The Chakra Handbook

Shalila Sharamon and Bodo J. Baginski

The Chakra Handbook

From a basic understanding
to practical application

A comprehensive guide to harmonizing
the energy centers with music, colors, gemstones,
scents, breathing techniques, reflex zone massage,
aspects of nature and meditation

1st English edition 1991
by Lotus Light Publications
P.O. Box 2
Wilmot, WI 53192, U.S.A.
The Shangri-La series is published
in cooperation with Schneelöwe Verlagsberatung,
Federal Republic of Germany
© 1988 reserved by Windpfered Verlagsgesellschaft m.b.H., Aitrang,
Federal Republic of Germany
All rights reserved
Translated by Peter Hübner
Edited by Judith Harrison, Munich
Cover design by Wolfgang Jünemann,
using a color drawing by Shalila Sharamon
Illustrations by Klaus-Peter Hüsch

ISBN 0-941524-85-X
Printed in the USA

Contents

Words of Introduction

At some point in life, nearly every human being asks him or herself the question, "Who am I?", "Which powers work through me?", "What are the capabilities still hidden in my innermost being?", and "How can I realize my full potential for happiness and creativity?"

We believe that no other area of knowledge can answer these questions as thoroughly as the knowledge of the human energy centers, otherwise known as "chakras". In learning to understand the full scope of the chakras' purpose and way of functioning, we see gain insight into the potential of man for perfection, a potential which is so fascinating and noble that all we can do is stand in awe of the miracle of Creation.

The purpose of this book is to help you recognize and realize this inherent human potential.

In order to work with the chakras effectively, it is not necessary to possess clairvoyant gifts or powers of any sort. You will, however, notice that your sensitivity in regard to the subtle levels will increase remarkably. You will also come to an understanding that will unite fragments of knowledge and experience into a perfectly comprehensible harmonious whole.

The activation and harmonization of the chakras is so easy that at certain points along the path we gained the impression that the knowledge of them is wrapped in mystery simply to prevent people from underestimating its intrinsic value, and to ensure that it is passed on from one generation to the next by the initiated. The fact that so many of us today are able to grasp and understand this treasury of knowledge may be due to recent evolutionary advancement.

Besides describing the chakras themselves and ways of working with them, this book also provides a number of easily learned exercises for harmonizing these energy centers. The techniques were chosen in a constellation that will bring about a gentle revitalization of the chakras as well as dissolution of blockages. It matters little which of these methods you choose to implement. All that is important is that you start to do one of them, because it YOUR fulfillment that is at stake, your fulfillment in THIS life, here and now.

While you read this book and practise the therapies described, we hope you will feel as much love and respect for the laws of life as we were able to in the course of recognizing these interwoven relationships and formulating them for this book.

Shalila and Bodo J.

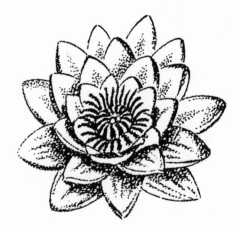

The Energy System and the Subtle Bodies

Most people consider the material world and the physical body to be the only reality that exists, as only these things can be discerned with the physical senses and grasped by the rational mind. In viewing a human being, however, the sensitized eye can perceive numerous energy structures, energy movements and shapes and colors within and around the physical body.

Should you be someone who only accepts the material body as reality, please consider what happens to the energy, the vital force which lends life to the physical body and provides it with sensations and means of expression when that body dies. A law of physics states that energy is never lost in the universe, it is merely transformed. The power at work behind the body's material appearance with all its functions and capabilities consists of a complex energy system without which the physical body could not exist. This system of energy consists of three basic components:

1. The subtle bodies, or energy bodies.
2. The chakras, or energy centers.
3. The *nadis*, or energy channels.

In this system, the *nadis* represent a kind of subtle network of arteries. The term *nadi* (pronounced nade-eye) is Sanskrit and means a pipe, vessel or vein. The function of a *nadi* is to transport *prana*, or vital energy, throughout man's subtle energy system.

The Sanskrit word *prana* may be translated as "absolute energy". In the Chinese and Japanese realm this universal life energy is called "chi", "ki" or "qi". It represents the primal source of all forms of energy and manifests itself in various frequencies. One of its forms of expression is air, which is one of several ways in which we take in *prana*, namely by breathing.

The level of consciousness of every living being depends on the frequencies of *prana* it is capable of absorbing and storing. Animals have lower frequencies than human beings, and advanced human beings have higher frequencies than those at the beginning of their development.

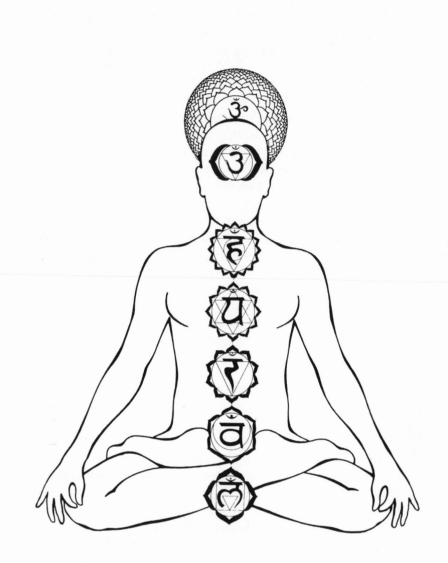

The *nadis* of one energy body are connected with the *nadis* of the neighboring energy body via the chakras. Some ancient Indian and Tibetan texts mention 72,000 *nadis*; other archaic writings speak of 350,000 *nadis*. The most important of these energy channels are called *sushumna*, *ida* and *pingala*, and will be treated in detail in the following chapter. The Chinese and Japanese speak of a similar system of energy channels, which they call meridians. (Acupuncture is based on knowledge of the meridians.)

The chakras, on the other hand, act as receivers, transformers and distributors of the various forms of *prana*. Through the *nadis* the chakras take up vital energy from man's subtle energy bodies, his surroundings, the cosmos and the basis of all manifestation, and transform them into the frequencies needed by the various areas of the physical or subtle bodies for their sustenance and development. Beyond this they give off energy into their surroundings. By means of this energy system the human being is therefore in a state of continual exchange with the powers at work at diverse levels of the environment, the universe, and Creation.

As the chakras operate in close interaction with the energy bodies, the characteristics and functions of these bodies are dealt with in this chapter. The individual chakras are described in detail in seven chapters, each one devoted to an individual chakra.

As a rule, there are said to be four energy bodies:

1. The ethereal body.
2. The emotional or astral body.
3. The mental body.
4. The spiritual or causative body.

Each of these bodies possesses its own fundamental vibrational frequency. The ethereal body, which is closest to the physical body, vibrates with the lowest frequency. The astral and mental bodies have higher frequencies and the spiritual body has the highest frequency of all.

Each of these bodies resembles a dance of energies within its individual frequency range, and as the human being advances in development, the respective frequencies rise accordingly. These bodies are the bearers of consciousness at their levels of vibration. When their vibrational frequency rises, they provide the human being with higher forms of vital energy, sensations and awareness.

The various energy bodies are not separate from one another. They pervade each other while continuing to vibrate in their individual frequency range and someone possessing the capability of seeing them can

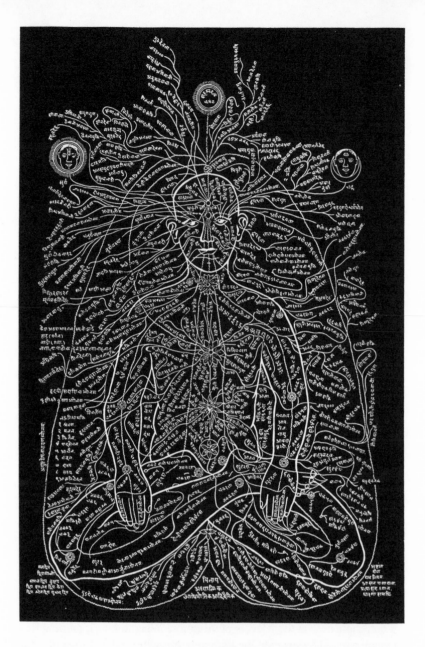

This illustration shows a historic depiction of a chakra and *nadi* chart from Tibet. Beside the seven main chakras we can see a large number of secondary chakras, as well as a complex network of subtle energy channels, the *nadis*. Some traditional text passages mention 350,000 *nadis* carrying cosmic energy. These *nadis* unite to form 14 main channels which in turn correspond to the main and secondary chakras.

differentiate between them if his vision is attuned to the specific sphere. If he wants to see the astral body, he will have to tune his vision to the astral sphere; if he wants to see the mental body, he will have to tune his vision to the mental sphere; and so on.

The Ethereal Body

The ethereal body resembles the physical body in shape and dimension, and is therefore sometimes called the "ethereal twin" or "inner physical body". It is the bearer of the powers that shape the physical body's, the vital, creative energy of life, and all physical sensation.

The ethereal body is formed anew with each reincarnation and dissolves within three to five days after physical death. (The astral, mental and spiritual bodies continue to exist after death and reunite with the newly formed physical body in every reincarnation.)

The ethereal body draws vital energies from the sun via the solar plexus chakra, and from the earth via the root chakra. It stores these energies and feeds them in continuous streams through the chakras and *nadis* into the physical body. These two forms of energy assure a living balance within the body's cells. When the organism's hunger for energy is stilled, the ethereal body lets off excess energy through the chakras and the pores of the skin. The energy leaving the pores exits in streams up to 2" in length, thus forming the ethereal aura that adepts usually see first as part of the aura as a whole. These rays envelop the physical body like a protective layer. They prevent disease-causing germs and harmful material from entering the body and simultaneously radiate a steady stream of vital energy into the environment.

This natural protection means that a person basically cannot fall ill from external causes. The causes of sickness always lie within. Negative thoughts and emotions as well as a lifestyle not in harmony with the natural needs of the body (stress, an unhealthy diet, excessive use of alcohol, nicotine and drugs) may use up the ethereal life force, leading to a lessening in the strength and intensity of energy radiation. In this manner the aura develops weak areas. The energy streams leaving the body appear bent rather than straight, or else cross each other in a disorderly manner. In this case the adept will see "holes" or "fissures" in the aura that may permit negative vibrations and disease-causing bacteria to enter the body. At the same time, vital energy may also "leak out" through these wounds in the subtle sheath.Because of the close relation-ship between the condition of the physical body and the energy radiation of the ethereal body, it is often referred to as a health aura. Therefore illness will become manifest up in the ethereal aura before becoming evident in the physical body. However, it can be recognized and treated at this level. This has been made possible by the process known as Kirlian photography, which makes this radiation of energy, which is inherent to every living being, visible on photographic paper.* Highly accurate diagnoses can be made on the basis of this invention, meaning that diseases can be recognized while still latent.

Both the ethereal body and physical body reacts strongly to thought impulses stemming from the mental body. This is the reason why positive thinking is successful in influencing health. By employing positive suggestions in a specific manner, we can readily enhance our body's health.

Another important function of the ethereal body is the role it plays as mediator between the higher energy bodies and the physical body in that it transfers information which we gain through our physical senses to the astral and mental bodies while simultaneously transporting energy and information from the higher bodies to the physical body. If the ethereal body is weakened, this transfer of energy and information will be impaired, and the person may appear to be emotionally and mentally indifferent.In order to harmonize and recharge the ethereal body, various forms of therapy are described in the latter part of this book.

In this context it is interesting to note that plants - especially flowers and trees - possess an energy radiation that is very similar to that given off by the human ethereal body. You may use this radiation to supply your own aura with renewed energy. This energy is also contained in ethereal oils, as described in a further chapter. You can also enter into direct connection with the energy of plants, however. In order to do this, sit down on the ground with your back against a tree of your liking, or embrace it in such a way that your entire body is in contact with it. Now simply permit the tree's energy-giving, harmonizing power to enter you. You could also try lying down on a meadow of fragrant blossom and letting the gentle vibrations of flowers envelop and pervade you. Even potted or cut flowers near you will gladly let you have some of their revitalizing, harmonizing energy. Plants react to your love and gratitude for this service by radiating even more energy, for it is one of their functions to help humans in this manner.

*This is a special high-frequency photography process developed by and named after the Russian scientists Semjon D. and Valentina K. Kirlian, his wife.

The Astral Body

The astral body, also know as the emotional body, is the carrier of feelings, emotions and character traits. It occupies about the same space as the physical body. In a hardly developed person, its contours are barely discernible and the astral body has the appearance of a cloud-like substance that moves about chaotically and in all directions. The higher developed a person is with regard to feelings, inclinations and character traits, the brighter and clearer the astral body will appear. In this case the adept will see clear-cut contours completely adapted to the shape of the physical body.

The aura of the astral body has an oval form and may extend several yards beyond and around the person. Every change in emotions is radiated out into the aura by the astral body. This takes place primarily through the chakras and to a small extent through the pores. The emotional aura is constantly in motion. Beside the fundamental and relatively steady character traits, which will be visible as constant, basic colors in the aura, the astral body also mirrors every momentary feeling, all fleeting emotions.

Thus the astral body consists of an indescribable play of constantly changing colors, shining in all imaginable hues. While emotions such as fear, anger, depression or worry will cause dark clouds to appear in the aura, the more a person opens up his or her consciousness to love, devotion and joy, the brighter and more transparent the colors of the emotional aura will glow.

None of the other subtle bodies shapes the average person's view of the world and reality as strongly as does the astral body. It stores all our unresolved emotions, conscious and unconscious fears and aggressions as well as feelings of loneliness, rejection and a lack of self-confidence, etc. These transmit their vibrations via the emotional aura and constitute the unconscious message passed on to the external world. At this point, the principle of mutual attraction comes into play. The energy vibrations which we send out attract the same vibrations from our environment and unite with them. This means that we are frequently confronted with precisely the people and circumstances that mirror what we are con-sciously avoiding or want to be rid of, or what we fear. In this way our environment serves us as a mirror which shows us all the elements we have banned from our consciousness into our subconscious. However, the unresolved feelings in our astral body are anxious to stay alive and if possible, to increase. And thus they lead us into situations time and time again that entail a repetition of the original emotional vibrations, for these vibrations form a source of nourishment for them.

If a person carries unresolved fear within him, he will frequently attract situations which confirm this very fear; if another harbors aggressions, for example, he will come across people who live out their anger and aggression again and again. For example, if we have resolved not to complain any more in certain situations without having resolved the basic aggression, it can very well happen that somebody in our vicinity will suddenly begin to holler at us.

Conscious thought and the intellectual goals of the mental body have little influence on the astral body, which follows its own laws. It can direct external behavior, but cannot override subconscious patterns.

Therefore a person may consciously strive for love and success and yet unconsciously radiate contradictory jealousy frequencies or lack in self-confidence, thus preventing him or herself from reaching their conscious goal.

If emotional problems are not resolved, they will continue to exist throughout successive incarnations, since the astral body survives physical death and joins the new physical body after reincarnation. The unresolved experiences stored in the astral body will also determine the conditions of the new life to a large extent.

Once we have fully understood these matters, we will have no other choice than to stop seeing ourselves as "victims" and making others or circumstances responsible for our weaknesses and misery. This realization in itself represents a considerable degree of liberation, for we now know that our destiny lies in our own hands, to a very great extent, and that we can change our lives by changing ourselves.

The majority of the "emotional knots" in the astral body are localized in the area of the solar plexus chakra. It is through this chakra that we react emotionally to direct experiences. If we wish, however, to recognize and become aware of our emotional patterns on a rational level, we have to employ the intuitive third eye chakra, the astral body's highest form of expression, to penetrate the contents of the solar plexus chakra. But even this will not entail true liberation. Emotional patterns of behaviour can only be resolved via the astral body, which expresses the wisdom, love and bliss of our Higher Self. At the same time, its holistic, universal character helps us recognize certain inner relationships. The connection to the astral body can be established via the heart and crown chakras.

The Higher Self does not condemn, it does not judge experiences to be "good" or "bad". It shows us that we go through certain experiences for the sole reason of learning to understand which feelings and actions result in a separation from the Divine Source and thereby cause suffering, and in order for us to grasp and understand the cosmic laws of natural balance. In tho areas of life in which we today experience ourselves as "victims", we were frequently the "perpetrator" in past incarnations.

In chakra therapy, an inner attitude that lets us accept the experiences and contents of the astral body and observe all the spontaneously appearing images and sensations without judging or rejecting any part of them is of greatest importance. In this manner our Higher Self can "take command" and let the spiritual energies of our highest energy bodies flow into our entire being.

When the vibrations of the spiritual body unite with the astral body and permeate it, the astral body begins to vibrate faster and faster, ridding itself of its stored negative experiences, as these have lower frequencies. Thus we lose the emotional memory of these experiences, enabling us to forgive ourselves and others.

The more these petrified emotional patterns are resolved, the more the astral body begins to radiate deep feelings of love and unconditional joy. The emotional aura glows in its clearest, brightest and most transparent of colors, and the messages it sends out to its environment attract love and happiness. An almost miraculous ability to cause everything it wishes for to happen is the natural result of a perfectly integrated astral body vibrating at its highest frequency-rate.

The Mental Body

Our thoughts, ideas and our rational and intuitive perceptions are all borne by the mental body. Its vibrations are higher than those of the ethereal and astral bodies and its structure is less dense. It is oval in shape, and as the person advances to a higher plane, its volume may increase to the point where it takes up about as much space as the astral body and the emotional aura combined. The aura radiation of the mental body exceeds these by several yards.

In the case of a mentally low-developed person, the mental body has the appearance of a milky white substance. Its few colors are muted and dull and its structure appears to be relatively impermeable. The more alive a person's thoughts are and his deeper awareness is, the clearer and more intensely the colors of the mental body will glow.

Just like the astral body, the mental body possesses both a higher and a lower octave. Its lower frequencies are expressed by the linear thinking of the rational mind, the approach adopted by most people to truth. This kind of mental activity is based on perceptions at the physical level, whereby information is taken on by the physical body and its senses and transferred to the astral body via the ethereal body. The astral body translates the information into feelings and passes them on to the mental body, which in turn reacts by formulating corresponding verbal thoughts. Through the influence of the astral body and its unresolved emotional patterns, the information is frequently distorted and thinking becomes biased. Repetitive thought patterns arise which are used by us to evaluate happenings in our world. This means that the rational mind can practically be never unbiased and neutral, although it claims this of itself.

Thoughts that arise in the mental body in this manner generally have to do with personal well-being and concerns regarding worldly matters. In this process the main function of the mental body is increasingly concerned with providing rational solutions to problems. This, however, is a distortion of its original character and a limitation of its capabilities. The function the mental body is actually meant to fulfill consists of taking up the universal truths reaching it from the plane of the spiritual body and integrating them with the rational mind. This, in turn, is meant apply these truths to concrete situations and bring about solutions in harmony with universal law.

The knowledge that comes to us in this manner from the spiritual plane of our being expresses itself in the form of intuition and sudden insights - such as images or sounds - that are then transformed into verbal thoughts. It gives us insight into the true nature of things and is holographic in nature, as opposed to the linear comprehension originating from the rational mind.

The higher octave of the mental body can be reached via a connection of the third eye chakra with the crown chakra.
Once the mental body is fully developed it becomes the mirror of the spiritual body, and the person realizes the wisdom and holistic cognition of the Higher Self in his life.

The Spiritual Body

The spiritual body, frequently referred to as the causative body, possesses the highest vibrational frequency of all the energy bodies. In human beings not yet highly conscious on the spiritual plane, its aura only extends to about a yard from the physical body. Compared to this, the spiritual aura of a totally awakened person can radiate outward for miles, with the original oval shape changing to a perfect circle.

If you have ever had the opportunity of being in the presence of an enlightened master, you may have noticed that the atmosphere suddenly changes when you are move more than a mile away. The experience of light, abundance and love which may fulfill you in a master's presence loses its intensity as soon as you leave the range of his aura.

The spiritual body and its aura glow in the gentlest of colors, which at the same time possess a deep radiance that cannot be described in words. The spiritual body constantly receives the highest, most radiant energy from the spiritual level of being. As this energy changes into successively lower frequencies, it also streams through the mental, astral and ethereal bodies. It accelerates the vibrations of these bodies and helps them to find the highest levels of expression in their own spheres. The extent to which we consciously perceive, absorb and use this energy depends on the corresponding development of the chakras.

Through the spiritual body we experience inner unity with all life. It connects us with pure Divine Being, the omnipresent basis of Creation from which all manifestation comes forth. By operating from this plane we gain inner access to all that exists in Creation.

The spiritual body is that divine part of us which is immortal, while the other subtle bodies slowly dissolve in the course of time as the person develops beyond the stages of consciousness necessitating existence on the worldly, astral and mental planes.

Only through our spiritual body is it possible to recognize the source and goal of our being and the purpose of our lives. When we open ourselves to its vibrations, our lives are enriched with a completely new quality. In all our actions we are borne by our Higher Self and our lives expresses wisdom, power, bliss and all-encompassing love, the natural characteristics of the highest aspect of our Self.

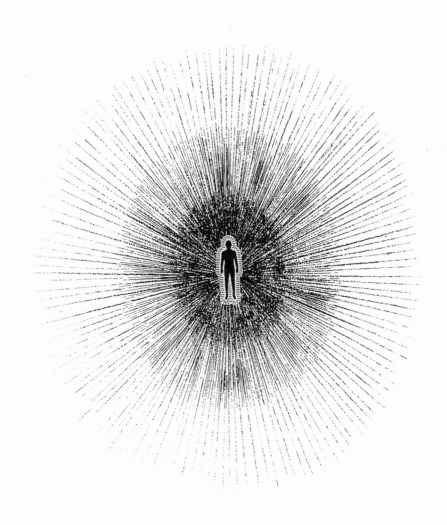

The human aura, beginning from the inside: 1) the ethereal aura; 2) the emotional
aura; 3) the mental aura; 4) the spiritual aura.

The Function and Purpose of the Chakras

In this chapter we would like to present you with the most important information on the way the chakras function. The theoretical understanding of these functions provides the foundation on which practical knowledge of the individual chakras is built up.

Traditional writings mention 88,000 chakras. This means that there is scarcely a minute area of the human body which is not a sensitive organ for the reception, transformation and transferral of energies. Most of these chakras are extremely small and only have a minor role to play in the energy system. Only approximately 40 secondary chakras can be considered significant. The most important of these are located in the area of the spleen, the back of the neck, the palms of the hands and the soles of the feet. The seven primary chakras, which are located along a central, vertical axis at the front of the body, are of such relevance for the functioning of the most important and fundamental aspects of the human body, mind and soul that we have devoted a separate chapter to each of them. Here you will find a description of the spiritual/mental characteristics assigned to each chakra, which areas of the body they influence, how they are affected by blockages, and much, much more.

For the moment we limit ourselves to a description of the characteristics common to all seven of the primary chakras. The true seat of the seven main chakras is in the ethereal body. They resemble funnel-shaped blossoms, each possessing a different number of petals, which is why they are often referred to as lotus blossoms in the East. The petals of the blossoms represent *nadis*, or energy channels, through which energy is able to flow into the chakras, where it is then conveyed to the subtle bodies. The number of petals, or *nadis*, ranges from four at the root chakra to nearly a thousand at the crown.

From the deepest point at the center of each chakra blossom, a stem-like channel extends to the spine and merges with it, connecting the chakras with the most important energy channel, the *sushumna*, which rises up within the spine to the top of the head.

The chakras are constantly in a state of rotation. This is why they are called "chakra", which in Sanskrit means "wheel". It is their rotating which attracts energy and draws it in or gives it off, depending on the direction of rotation.

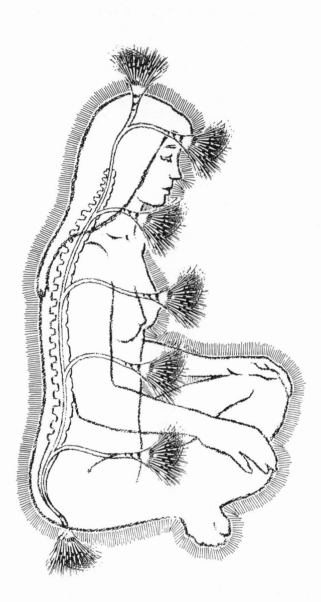

A side-view of the funnel-shaped chakras, their connection to the main channel in the spine, and the way they radiate out from the physical body.

The chakras rotate either to the right (clockwise) or to the left, depending on sex, thus enabling the energies of man and woman to complement each other. This is because the chakras that turn to the right in a man rotate in the opposite direction in a woman, and vice versa. Every clockwise rotation is primarily male, or, in accordance with Chinese teaching, Yang, in nature, meaning that it represents willpower and activity as well the more negative characteristics of aggression and force. Every counterclockwise rotation is female or Yin in nature, and represents receptiveness and agreement, as well as the more negative characteristic of weakness. The direction in which a chakra rotates varies from chakra to chakra. The male root chakra, for example, rotates to the right, expressing the characteristics of this center in the sense of conquering and mastering, both materially and sexually, while the female root chakra rotates to the left, making women more receptive for the stimulating and life-giving power of the earth flowing through the root center. In the second chakra the portents change: the woman's chakra now rotates to the right, indicating greater activity in the expression of emotions, while the man's second chakra turns to the left, indicating a tendency to receive on an emotional level or frequently remain passive. And so it continues: the rotations alternate, thus shaping men and women in different ways and leading to supplementation of energies in every area of life.

Knowledge of the rotational direction of the chakras can play a role in several forms of therapy. When using aroma therapy, for instance, you may wish to apply fragrances in circular movements corresponding to the chakra, or, if you are working with gemstones, you can again follow the direction of the energy center in question.

Most people's chakras extend about 4" in all directions from their point of origin. Each of the energy centers contains all color vibrations, although one particular color always dominates, corresponding to the primary task of the chakra. With the advancing development of a person, the chakras extend out further and the frequency of their vibrations increases. Additionally, their colors also become clearer and brighter.

The size and vibration rate of the chakras determine the amount and quality of the energies they are able to absorb from various sources. These are energies that come to us from the cosmos, the stars and nature, from all things and people in our environment, our different subtle bodies and the non-manifest basis of all being. These energies partially reach the chakras via the *nadis*, but they also flow into them directly.

The two most important and fundamental forms of energy enter the human system via the root center and the crown center. These two chakras are connected by the *sushumna*, which in turn is connected to the chakras

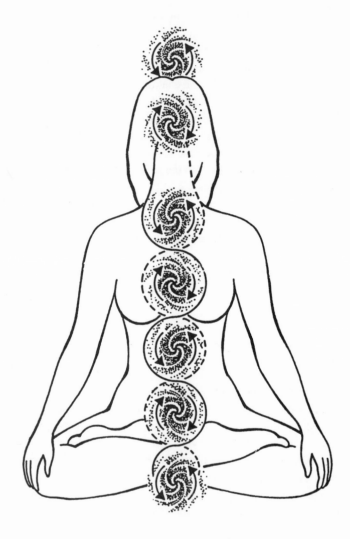

The uninterrupted line spiralling up to the head represents *pingala*, or solar energy, while the dotted line symbolizes *ida*, or lunar energy.

The direction of the chakras in men

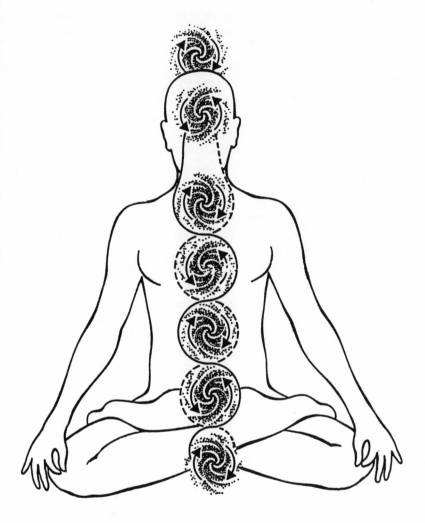

The uninterrupted line spiralling up to the head represents *pingala*, while the dotted line symbolizes *ida*.

via "stems" along which it provides them with vital energy. At the same time, the *sushumna* is also the channel through which the so-called *kundalini* power rises. The *kundalini* power rests at the lower end of the spine "rolled up like a snake" and enters the system through the root center. It represents the creative cosmic energy which is also referred to as Shakti in Indian teachings, the female expression of God. This aspect of Divine Being brings forth all manifestation in Creation. Its opposite is the pure, unformed aspect of Divine Being resting in itself, which we shall discuss in greater detail further on.

In most people, the *kundalini* power flows through the *sushumna* in a mere trickle. When it is awakened by growing consciousness, however, it rises up the *sushumna* as a swelling stream, and activates the chakras. This activation causes the energy centers to expand and speeds up their frequencies. In other words, *kundalini* supplies the chakras with the vibrations that man has needed during the course of his evolution in order to gain various energetic and material capabilities and integrate them into his life.

As *kundalini* rises, its energy is transformed into a different vibration in each of the chakras, in each case corresponding to the purpose of the chakra in question. The vibration is lowest in the root center and has its highest form of expression in the crown center. The transformed vibrations are passed on to the different subtle bodies and the physical body, and are perceived as feelings, thoughts and physical sensations.

The degree to which a person permits to work within him depends on the degree of consciousness he has attained in the various areas of life represented by the various chakras, and whether they are blocked by stress and unresolved experiences. The more conscious a person is, the more active and open his chakras will be, and the more *kundalini* will be able to enter them as a strong stream. The more this occurs, the more active the chakras become in turn, leading to a further increase in consciousness. In this way, as we begin to remove the blockages to our chakras and follow the path towards developing consciousness, we set in motion a steady cycle of action and reaction.

Besides *kundalini* energy there is also another power which flows through the spine to each individual chakra. It is the energy of pure divine Being, the unmanifested aspect of God, the energy which enables the human being to recognize the unformed aspect of Divine Being as the unchangeable and omnipresent basis of all levels of manifestation. This energy, which enters the body through the crown chakra, is especially suited for dissolving blockages within the chakras. In the archaic teachings of India it is known as the god Shiva, the great destroyer of

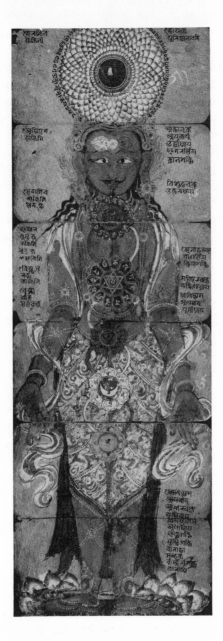

This Nepalese depiction of the chakras is approximately 350 years old. The lotus blossoms depict the seven primary chakras, which represent levels of consciousness that become finer and finer, the higher they are to be found in the body. The most important energy channels, *sushumna*, *ida* and *pingala*, can also be seen. (Gouache on paper.)

ignorance whose mere presence initiates a transformation towards the Divine.

Thus Shiva and Shakti work hand in hand in the holistic development of the human being, in a development in which the Divine is integrated into our lives in the same way as all levels of relative being.

Beside the *sushumna*, there are two additional energy channels, known in Sanskrit as *ida* and *pingala*, that play particularly important roles in the energy system. *Pingala* functions as the carrier of solar energy, which is full of heat and drive. This channel begins on the right hand side of the root chakra and ends in the upper area of the right nostril. *Ida* is the carrier of cool and calming lunar energy. Its channel begins left of the root chakra and ends in the left nostril. On their way up from the root chakra to the nose both these *nadis* wind themselves around the *sushumna*.

Ida and *pingala* are able to take *prana* directly from the air via our breath, and discharge toxic matter when we breathe out. Together with the *sushumna* they represent the three main channels of the energy system. The secondary chakras and the subtle energy bodies provide the chakras with energy via a large number of *nadis*, which also transfer energy from the chakras themselves to the energy bodies.

The chakras also take up direct vibrations from the environment when these correspond to their individual frequencies. By acting as antennas for the entire range of energy vibrations, they connect us with what is going on in our environment, in nature and in the universe. Thus the chakras can be seen as subtle sensory organs. Our physical body, equipped as it is with senses, is a vehicle adjusted to the laws of life on our planet. It enables us to find our way in the outer aspects of life, while helping us to realize and put to use our inner values as well as the knowledge gained on this earth. In this respect, the chakras act as receivers of the energy vibrations and information transcending the physical realm. They are the openings that connect us with the unlimited world of subtle energies.

The chakras also radiate energy directly into our environment and thus change the atmosphere in our vicinity. Through the chakras we can send out healing vibrations as well as conscious or subconscious messages that influence people, situations and even matter, both in a positive and in a negative sense.

In order to experience wholeness and the creativity, knowledge, strength, love and bliss this entails, the chakras have to be open and work together harmoniously. This is the case with very few people. As a rule, the individual chakras are activated at different degrees, especially the two lower ones. Indeed, in persons of prominent social standing or holding a position of great influence, the solar plexus chakra is often disproportionally active. At the same time, there also exist every conceivable combination of open, blocked or one-sidedly active chakras. These states also undergo change during the course of a lifetime, since basic themes are always moving to the foreground and withdrawing again.

For this reason, knowledge of the chakras can be of immeasurable help in getting to know yourself, can guide you in the realization of your inherent potential and enable you to live a life full of abundance and joy.

Human Development Cycles in the Light of the Chakra Teachings

Everything in our universe is subject to specific rhythms and cycles. This begins at the level of the atoms and encompasses all forms of being in Creation. Fixed, rhythmic laws can be seen everywhere - in our heartbeat and in respiration, in the alternation of day and night, in the coming and going of the seasons and in the predictable movement of the stars. Cycles also repeat themselves in the development of living creatures. For example, in the case of a plant we can observe how first the sprout appears, then the first leaves, later the bud and the flower, to be followed by the fruit. A certain sequence of stages is always maintained. It is therefore logical that the human being, a spiritual entity in a material body, also develops according to a certain sequence. The human being does not merely grow older every day and gain additional skills and experiences, its development also takes place according to special mental and spiritual cycles. A certain theme or subject will not carry the same weight in every stage of life, and on examining this fact more closely we soon recognize that "Mother Nature" confronts us with specific tasks at certain times that have to be absolved precisely then. Even though these tasks appear in different guises, certain stages of development can only be realized to an optimal degree when carried out at specific phases of life. At the age of 25, for instance, it is very difficult to catch up on the development we should have experienced at the age of 5 or 12. This is the reason why the "house of life" always stands on a shaky foundation for some people, simply because certain experiences were not gained or skills not developed when they were at the right age for them.

The knowledge to be described here regarding life cycles is not new - it has simply been lost for a while. However, various schools of spiritual thought still include it in their teachings on the overall development of human beings. In anthroposophical circles, especially within the teaching methods of Rudolf Steiner, this knowledge is applied with regard to the natural development cycles in children. Rudolf Steiner, founder of the anthroposophical movement, wrote extensively on the subject. In the anthroposophical view, human life consists of clearly-segmented cycles divided into periods of seven years each. Different times are apparently marked by different qualities, that is to say, at certain times in life the human being is open to certain influences and experiences and is at this point mature enough for very specific steps in development.

It is interesting to note that this insight fits in perfectly with our knowledge of the function and purpose of the chakra system. We pass through a chakra every seven years, starting out with the root center, and the characteristics of the chakra in question become the base theme of our lives for the seven-year period. This seven-year period, however is divided up again into seven one-year periods, each corresponding to one of the seven chakras and stating out with the root center.

After the first seven-year period (characterized by the root chakra), we pass into the second seven-year period, this time characterized by the solar plexus chakra. And so we pass through successive stages of development, year after year, each year characterized by both the base theme in question and the individual one-year themes. After five seven-year periods we have more or less reached the middle of our lives, and after seven such periods we have completed an entire cycle. In other words, a completely new stage of life begins with our 50th birthday, giving us the chance to start all over again, but this time from a "higher octave" of development. From the 50th year on, very special lessons wait to be learned. People who reach the age of 98 have completed their second cycle of development.

Each year a new theme awaits us, and every seven years a new base theme, and in all cases they augment each other perfectly. Knowledge of the significance and purpose of each chakra can help us utilize every single year in a manner helpful for our development. Beyond that helps us understand the development of our children more fully and enables us to give them the kind of attention and stimulation they need at the right times.

A change also takes place on a material level every seven years. As you may know, it is a biological fact that our bodies renew themselves every seven years. In other words, after seven years all our body's cells have been replaced by new ones, and biologically speaking we are a completely new person. If we have the impression that nothing much has changed on the psychic plane, however, the reason will be that the astral body is still burdened with the patterns that existed at the beginning of the time segment. On the other hand, you may meet someone again after a long time and note with surprise that he or she has made a tremendous advance. A fundamental change within seven years is perfectly possible. We have provided a number of condensed tables on the following pages

Cycles of Human Development in the Light of Chakra Teachings
Age 1 - 49

	1st chakra	2nd chakra	3rd chakra	4th chakra	5th chakra	6th chakra	7th chakra
Main theme for one year							
	Primordial life energy and trust. Relationship to the earth and to the material world. Stability, power to achieve.	Primordial feelings, flowing with life, sensuality, eroticism, creativity, awe and enthusiasm.	Unfolding one's personality. Assimilation of feelings and experiences, shaping one's being. Influence and power, strength and abundance, wisdom growing out of experience.	Unfolding of the qualities of the heart, love, compassion, sharing, sincere involvement, selflessness, devotion and healing.	Communication, creative self-expression, being open. Expanse, independence, inspiration, access to the subtler levels of being.	Functions of realization. Intuition, development of the inner senses, mind power, projection of the will, manifestation.	Perfection, enlightenment through inner contemplation. Unity with the omnipresent being, universal consciousness.
	1st year	2nd year	3rd year	4th year	5th year	6th year	7th year
	8th year	9th year	10th year	11th year	12th year	13th year	14th year

Base theme for
a seven-year segment

1st chakra: age 1 - 7
Primordial life energy and trust.
Relationship to the earth and to
the material world. Stability,
power to achieve.

2nd chakra: age 8 - 14
Primordial feelings, flowing with
life, sensuality, eroticism, creativity, awe and enthusiasm.

3rd chakra: age 15 - 21. Unfolding one's personality. Assimilation of feelings and experiences, shaping one's being. Influence and power, strength and abundance, wisdom growing out of experience.	15th year	16th year	17th year	18th year	19th year	20th year	21st year
4th chakra: age 22 - 28. Unfolding of the qualities of the heart, love, compassion, sharing, sincere involvement, selflessness, devotion and healing.	22nd year	23rd year	24th year	25th year	26th year	27th year	28th year
5th chakra: age 29 - 35. Communication, creative self-expression, being open. Expanse, independence, inspiration, access to the subtler levels of being.	29th year	30th year	31st year	32nd year	33rd year	34th year	35th year
6th chakra: age 36 - 42. Functions of realization. Intuition, development of the inner senses, mind power, projection of the will, manifestation.	36th year	37th year	38th year	39th year	40th year	41st year	42nd year
7th chakra: age 43 - 49. Perfection, enlightenment through inner contemplation. Unity with the omnipresent being, universal consciousness.	43rd year	44th year	45th year	46th year	47th year	48th year	49th year

The human cycles of development in the light of the chakra teachings "Higher Octave", age 50 - 98

Main theme for one year

1st chakra	2nd chakra	3rd chakra	4th chakra	5th chakra	6th chakra	7th chakra
Primordial life energy and trust. Relationship to the earth and to the material world. Stability, power to achieve.	Primordial feelings, flowing with life, sensuality, eroticism, creativity, awe and enthusiasm.	Unfolding one's personality. Assimilation of feelings and experiences, shaping one's being. Influence and power, strength and abundance, wisdom growing out of experience.	Unfolding of the qualities of the heart, love, compassion, sharing, sincere involvement, selflessness, devotion and healing.	Communication, creative self-expression, being open. Expanse, independence, inspiration, access to the subtler levels of being.	Functions of realization. Intuition, development of the inner senses, mind power, projection of the will, manifestation.	Perfection, enlightenment through inner contemplation. Unity with the omnipresent being, universal consciousness.
50th year	51st year	52nd year	53rd year	54th year	55th year	56th year
57th year	58th year	59th year	60th year	61st year	62nd year	63rd year

Base theme for
a seven-year segment

1st chakra: age 50 - 56
Primordial life energy and trust.
Relationship to the earth and to
the material world. Stability,
power to achieve.

2nd chakra: age 57 - 63
Primordial feelings, flowing with
life, sensuality, eroticism, creativity, awe and enthusiasm.

3rd chakra: age 64 - 70	Unfolding one's personality. Assimilation of feelings and experiences, shaping one's being. Influence and power, strength and abundance, wisdom growing out of experience.	64th year	65th year	66th year	67th year	68th year	69th year	70th year
4th chakra: age 71 - 77	Unfolding of the qualities of the heart, love, compassion, sharing, sincere involvement, selflessness, devotion and healing.	71st year	72nd year	73rd year	74th year	75th year	76th year	77th year
5th chakra: age 78 - 84	Communication, creative self-expression, being open. Expanse, independence, inspiration, access to the subtler levels of being.	78th year	79th year	80th year	81st year	82nd year	83rd year	84th year
6th chakra: age 85 - 91	Functions of realization. Intuition, development of the inner senses, mind power, projection of the will, manifestation.	85th year	86th year	87th year	88th year	89th year	90th year	91st year
7th chakra: age 92 - 98	Perfection, enlightenment through inner contemplation. Unity with the omnipresent being, universal consciousness.	92nd year	93rd year	94th year	95th year	96th year	97th year	98th year

which show you what a person can expect to experience each year, and the influences he will be especially susceptible to. In the chapter that follows a number of examples are then explained in detail.

In ages past, the number seven was frequently used to denote completion, abundance and (spiritual) perfection. In many cultures it was regarded as a sacred number, and so even today we often come across the seven in religious writings, myths and fairy tales. The week also consists of a cycle of seven days. This is the ever-returning basic rhythm of our being. In the course of the Cultural Revolution, Mao Tse-tung, China's great leader, attempted to replace the seven-day week with one lasting ten days. The number of workers reporting sick took on such proportions a short while later, that China returned to the seven-day week.

It may be of interest to know that even before we are born we go through the various chakra stages. This development takes place in reversed order, however, beginning with the crown chakra, through which energetic light streams flow into the embryo throughout the entire prenatal phase. Following the development of the third eye chakra, the other chakras follow until at the end of pregnancy the root chakra finally develops - connecting the new human being with the world and preparing it to enter our atmosphere.

You may accept such laws as being real or not - whichever way, you will not affect the universal forces governing these laws, and while we are free to make decisions as we will, we nevertheless live within the framework of certain laws. So it is up to us whether we apply this knowledge or not.

Please Note: When consulting the tables on the phases of human development, please remember that you are always a year ahead of your year of birth, i.e. when you are "officially" 24 years old, you are actually 25, or when you when you have passed your 38th birthday, you are actually in your 39th year on this earth.

How Blockages Develop in the Chakras

Our true nature is to be one with the power which manifests itself in the endless array of vibrations and laws, colors and shapes, scents and sounds of all Creation. There is nothing we are separate from. The innermost core of our being lives in indivisible unity with the absolute, unchanging, omnipresent Being we call God, that which brought forth and permeates all areas of relative existence. According to its nature, this pure, unlimited being is bliss.

As soon as the still ocean of Divine Being resting in itself rises in waves of joy, the dance of Creation begins of which we, too, are an expression and in which we take part through our subtle and physical bodies.

Our awareness of this unity was lost in that moment in time when we as individuals began to rely solely on the information reaching us through our physical senses and rational mind, and thereby forgot our Divine origins. A separation seemed to occur, bringing about a very real experience of fear in its wake. We lost our feeling of inner fulfillment and security in life and began to seek it in our surroundings, but they disappointed our yearning for perfect fulfillment again and again. This experience caused the fear of new disappointments to arise. In the process we forgot that we can never be destroyed, that death is merely a changing of exterior form.

Fear invariably triggers a drawing together, a contraction or cramp which in turn increases the feeling of separateness and fear. To break out of this vicious circle and regain the lost sense of unity is the declared goal of practically all spiritual paths in the East and West.

The chakras are the relays in the human energy system that are the most susceptible to the forming of blockages arising from fear. Additional blockages also occur along the *nadis*. A permanent state of contraction can prevent the life energies from flowing freely and supplying our various bodies with all they need to mirror and maintain the consciousness of unity. When our experience of separation, of having been left alone, of inner emptiness and fear of death, causes us to seek in the exterior world those things that we can only find in the innermost core of our being, we make ourselves dependent on the love and recognition of others, physical sensations and success and material possessions. Instead of enriching our lives, these things become necessities with which we attempt to fill the void. If we lose them, we are suddenly confronted with nothingness, and that sneaking feeling of fear which accompanies practically every one of use through life suddenly stands before us again. And of course, it is the others who take away what we so obviously need for our fulfillment and satisfaction. We forget that we all have our common origin in the Divine Being and that on this level we are all part of one another. Instead of loving the people around us, we begin to see them as competitors or even as enemies. Finally we reach the point where we feel that we have to protect ourselves and prevent certain people, situations or information from getting too close. We withdraw our antennas to avoid having to face challenges and thereby cause further contractions in our chakras.

Yet our need for recognition by the people around us or by a group that we feel we belong to is so strong that we are prepared to change our lives to meet the expectations of these people or generally accepted social rules and repress our spontaneous feelings as soon as they no longer fit into the framework of social conventions. The only way we can do this is to draw our chakras together to such a degree that uncontrolled emotions can no longer pass the filter. This means that the energy in the chakra in question is dammed up. And because the energies can no longer be radiated out in their original form, they become distorted, break through the barrier anyway and discharge themselves in the form of strong and often negative emotions or an exaggerated need for activity.

This corresponds to a predominantly Yang reaction to the blockage. As it involves the expression of energy, however, new energy is able to move in, to be discharged again and again in the same inappropriate way.

A predominantly Yin reaction to the blockage of the chakras expresses itself as an almost total holding back of the energies. To a large extent this can almost completely halt the flow of energy, because no room is made for the energy moving up. The result is an inadequate supply of vital energy and a weakening of the afflicted chakra. The effects of impaired functioning as well as overloading are described in the chapters on the individual chakras. Your individual reactions may differ from the information provided since they are determined by personal experiences which caused the blockage in the first place and which are now stored in the astral body and, to a lesser degree, in the mental body.

These stored experiences are not left behind when physical death occurs. We take them with us from one incarnation to the next until we have resolved them in the course of our development. To a large degree they determine the circumstances into which we are born and the experiences that we unconsciously attract in our new life through the astral body.

However, during the childhood phase of each life we are given the opportunity of dissolving such emotional patterns very quickly. In the newborn person the entire energy system is completely permeable and open. This means that in principle every reborn soul is given the chance of leading a fulfilled life. But is also means that it is open for all vibrations and experiences and therefore for every kind of impression.

A newly-born human being cannot consciously shape its own life, nor can it talk about its experiences. It is therefore completely dependent on the good will and care of adults. This presents the parents with a great opportunity and an equally great task.

On the following pages we would like to describe the influences that a child needs in the first years of its life in order to develop well, to avoid new blockages and help resolve old patterns.

In this day and age many highly-developed souls are waiting for a suitable set of parents with whom they can incarnate without incurring unnecessary blockages that will hinder the completion of their tasks on earth. Other souls would like to be reborn into this age of change because such an opportunity for learning and growth will hardly present itself ever again.

The following knowledge can be of help to parents-to-be in providing the best possible start to a soul that would like to come to them as their child. It can also help each of us to understand our own "history of blockages" better and thus help us to resolve them more easily.

As a fetus experiences and perceives its world mostly through its mother, the beginnings of blockages in the energy system can start up in the womb if the life growing there feels rejected or the mother lives in a continual state of stress. Loving attention to the small being in the womb will provide its energy system with the vibrations that make it feel perfectly well and secure. If the mother experiences the months of her pregnancy as a happy and fulfilled time, she will be providing her child with the very best prerequisites for a happy and creative life.

The moment of birth is a milestone in the life of every human being, and can leave an impression that lasts a lifetime in that it can determine whether we perceive the world as a friendly and pleasant place or as hard, cold and lacking in love. At birth the child leaves the perfect physical security that provided it with nourishment and protection during the happy state of timelessness and weightlessness for the first nine months of its life on earth. Nonetheless, the little being is prepared for birth and is also curious about the world. Therefore a natural birth, during which mother and child are not weakened by medication, is not a shock to the child, although it means a great deal of effort and work. What it is not in the least prepared for is separation from the mother immediately after the birth. As long as it feels the accustomed vibrations of the mother's body and remains embedded within the energy vibrations of the aura it is used to, it is willing to open itself to new experiences in a feeling of trust.

Beyond this, bodily contact between mother and child immediately after birth establishes bonding. A stream of loving emotions and positive energy flows automatically and without conscious effort from the mother to the newborn child and continues without interruption as long as her body feels the baby near her or at least retains it in her emotional aura. This flow of love fills the little soul with trust and joy. It is interesting to note that fathers also develop more intimate feelings towards their babies and greater intuitive understanding when they are present at the moment of birth and are permitted to touch and hold the baby.

If the newborn is removed from the mother straight away after birth, it will experience a deep pain of separation and loneliness. As long as the mother can consciously send the newborn child her loving feelings and thoughts, contact is maintained between them and the child is not totally cut off from the mother's energy supply. If the mother becomes preoccupied with other things, however, or is fatigued and emotionally drained due to the medication she has received, this ongoing contact will be disrupted.

The newborn child will become aware of its helplessness in an unknown, cold world in which it feels completely alone without the protective, warming presence of its mother. This experience is so overpowering that as a rule the child's energy system is unable to cope with these frightening feelings and a deep impression is made, resulting in the first blockage of energies.

This blockage manifests itself primarily in the area of the root chakra. In the previous chapter we discussed life rhythms in the light of the chakra teachings. As you can see in the tables, the seven-year base theme and the one-year main theme deal with the energies of the root chakra during the first year of life. Beside the mastery of the physical and the material world, which has its initial high point in upright carriage towards the end of the first year, the development of primordial trust stands in the foreground at this time. This primordial trust forms the foundation for a person's overall potential to completely unfold without fear. At the same time, all the other centers are provided with the life energy of *kundalini* power via the root chakra. Thus a blockage in the root chakra will effect the entire energy system. It is by no means coincidental that psychologists consider the first year of a person's life the most important one of all. During this time, the child mainly gathers experience through its physical body, meaning that it needs bodily contact with its mother most of all, and with its father and other trusted individuals.

At this age a child has no sense of time. If it cries because it is lonely or hungry, it does not know if this condition will ever end and can easily fall into despair. If its needs are quickly satisfied, however, it develops the trusting feeling that this earth supplies its children with everything they require to maintain their bodies and satisfy their emotional needs. On the physical and subtle planes the child is able to open itself to the nourishing and protecting energies held ready for it by the mother planet.

Nearly all peoples still living close to nature possess intuitive knowledge about these processes. They constantly carry their infants close to their bodies and do not rest them elsewhere, even when the steady rocking motion has let them drift off into sleep. When the child reaches the crawling stage they will always pick it up and carry it around if this is what it wants. At night the children lie next to the mother, and if they feel hungry, the mother's breast is there. The sparkling eyes and satisfied expressions of these small human beings speak for themselves. The children of these peoples rarely cry and are prepared at an early age to take on social responsibility.

If a mother in our society devotes herself to caring for her child in such a manner for at least the first year, and is willing to disregard her own needs for that time, she will have provided it with the best possible potential for the rest of its life. We believe that this is really a worthwhile investment. The automatic flow of love and joy the mother experiences as a result of the constant bodily contact with her child is in itself abundant compensation for the many small things she may not be able to do during this time.

If a child loses the feeling of primordial trust, security, fulfillment and sheltering during this time, it will seek these things more and more in the external, material world as it grows older. It will establish relationships with things instead of people. This begins with cuddly toy animals that have to take the place of human warmth and closeness. Later on the child demands increasingly more toys and sweets in its unconscious search for something that will fill its nagging feeling of emptiness. Once it has reached adulthood, the fancy clothes, the car, the furnishings, the house and professional or social status become the things it clings to in order to regain the feeling of security and fulfillment lost in childhood. Our materialistic society, geared as it is to consumption, could not exist without the unsatisfied needs of the majority of its members.

But the number of people who realize that the experience of inner security and satisfaction cannot be attained through material goods is increasing. They are setting out on an inner search which actually is their only chance of rediscovering the lost paradise which most of us left at birth.

In the second year of life a new theme is added to the seven-year base theme of the root chakra. As it grows older the child establishes contact with the energies of the second chakra. The tender touches and affectionate hugging take on a significance beyond mere physical contact. The child begins to discover its sensuality and to experience and express its sensations and emotions more consciously. At this point the contents of the astral body, carried over from past lives, begin to gradually appear. In its second year the child initially experiences very basic emotional patterns.

It is now increasingly important that parents do not attempt to force certain attitudes on the child, because if they do it will begin to hold back emotions and remain in a rigid, given form. If, on the other hand, the child learns to simply experience its emotions, to accept their existence and deal with them playfully, it can dissolve all the negative emotional impressions in short order.

The parents should understand that a child does not express negativity at this age. If it is angry, then only for the reason that a natural need was disappointed. Angry crying or beating dissolves the blockage that has set in and frees the child from it. Yet most parents find it difficult to completely accept their child's expression of emotions, as they do not express their own. They love their child when it does this and avoids that and thereby give it to understand, "You are not good enough the way you are."

The child adopts the attitude of judging from the parents, and since it does not want to lose their love, pushes aside the unloved parts in itself. This has far-reaching energetic consequences. If sensual stimulation is lacking in addition to this, a deficiency of primordial trust in the emotional area will result and the sacral chakra will be blocked.

The adult then has difficulty accepting and expressing his natural emotions. In order to feel anything at all he requires coarse, sensual stimuli and develops a tendency to view others as objects that serve his satisfaction.

In its third year the little human being establishes contact with the energies of the solar plexus chakra. Emotional expression becomes more differentiated and what we said about the second year applies even more so. The child now wants to test itself as an individual personality, wants to get to know its own influence and says "no" time and time again in order to see what happens.

If a fight for power is taking place between parents and child because the parents think the only way they can raise the child is to force it to accept their will, this battle will reach its first climax during the child's third year. If the child with its awakening personality does not feel loved and accepted, the energies of the solar plexus chakra will be blocked. Once grown up, it will lack the confidence and courage to live its own personality, to shape its life according to its own ideas and to learn from negative experiences. Instead, it will conform or attempt to control the world around it.

And so the journey of the small human being continues through the energies of the various chakras. We feel that the examples given are adequate enough. The tables combined with the descriptions of the individual chakras will enable you to chart the remainder of the way yourself.

When we read these detailed explanations, we should always remember that we were the one who chose the circumstances of our reincarnation. We decided to join a certain set of parents in order to be filed into shape, to gather the experiences which our soul needs so that it can develop towards perfection.

Hardly any of us probably happened upon parents possessing such deep understanding and so much selfless love that in their loving and knowing hands the final limiting patterns of the astral body melted away. All this means is that it is our task and purpose in life to develop the understanding love towards ourselves that eliminates the blockages in us and resolves those unloved and disowned aspects of our soul. Without being conscious of it, our parents are our first teachers, for through their reactions to our behavior they sometimes make us painfully aware of our shortcomings and thus provide us with the impetus to find a way of restoring the lost feeling of inner wholeness. Later on in life, other people and situations that we have purposely yet unconsciously attracted take over this task, serving as mirrors for those parts of our soul that we have consigned into the shadowy areas of our psyche.

In the following chapter we will now be discussing means of eliminating chakra blockages that will help you find the way back to the experience of inner wholeness.

Eliminating Blockages

There are two fundamental ways of influencing our chakras in a harmonious and liberating manner. The first way consists of exposing the chakras to energy vibrations that are close to the ones in which a harmoniously functioning chakra free of blockages naturally vibrates. Such energy vibrations can be found in pure, glowing colors, in gemstones, in sounds and ethereal oils as well as in the elements and the profusion of expression found in nature. The practical application of all of these means is described in the therapy chapter of this book.

As soon as frequencies flow into the chakras that are higher and purer than the energies present in the chakra itself, they begin to vibrate faster, and the slower frequencies of the blockages dissolve step by step. New vital energies can now be absorbed by the energy centers and be passed on to the subtle bodies without hindrance. It is as if a fresh breeze were blowing through our energy system. The prana streaming in provides the ethereal body with energy, which it in turn passes on to the physical body. The energy flows into the astral body and the mental body, dissolving blockages here, too, since the vibrations of these bodies are slower that those of the inflowing energy. Finally, the nadis of the entire energy system pulse with vital energy, and body, mind and soul begin to vibrate on a higher plane and radiate with health and joy.

When the dammed up energies are set free during this process of cleansing and purification, their contents once again enter our consciousness. We can experience once more the same feelings that caused the blockage in the first place - our fears, our anger and our pain. Bodily ills may come to the surface one last time before being cleared up completely. While this is going on, we may feel unsettled, irritable or extremely tired. As soon as the channels are cleared for the intake of energy, a deep feeling of joy, serenity and clarity enters us.

But many people do not have the courage to undergo the necessary process of purification. They often lack the knowledge needed and interpret the returning experiences as a regression in their development. The fact is that the blockages in our energy system will only be eliminated to the extent that our overall development permits us to take a close look at the unloved and suppressed parts of our Self and redeem them with our love. This brings us to the second method mentioned at the outset of this chapter. Although it should always accompany the method of direct activation and cleansing of the chakras, it represents a separate means of harmonizing our entire energy system and freeing it from blockages.

This method has as its aim the achievement of an inner attitude of unconditional acceptance, leading in turn to complete relaxation. Relaxation is the opposite of and remedy for anxiety, cramping up and blockages. As long as we consciously or unconsciously deny any area in ourselves, as long as we judge ourselves and thereby condemn and reject parts of ourselves, we maintain a state of tension which prevents complete relaxation and the elimination of blockages.

Time and time again we have met people who said they just could not relax. Even in their leisure time or while on vacation these people constantly need diversion or activity, and if ever they actually seem to rest, their inner dialogue does not stop. As soon as they calm down externally, they feel an inner unrest. The self-healing mechanism is so active in these people, however, that their blockages begin to dissolve as soon as their energy system is able to calm down a bit. But since they do not understand this mechanism, they constantly flee into activity and thereby suppress the resolving and cleansing of the blocked energies.

Other people isolate themselves in their mental body in order to avoid the confrontation with the contents of their astral body. With these people all experience takes place via the mind. They analyze, interpret and categorize, but never enter into an experience with their entire being.

Occasionally we have also met people trying to force an opening of the chakras, for instance by practising certain *kundalini* yoga exercises in excess and without proper guidance, only to be swamped by the subconscious contents of the chakra in question. And in the attempt to force these contents back, new and even deeper blockages can be created. Occasionally someone travelling a spiritual path will only activate his or her higher chakras because he or she unconsciously does not wish to identify with the contents of the lower chakras should they be set free. Such a person may gain wonderful experiences from the realm of the higher chakras, and yet feel a lack or deficiency deep inside. Unconditional joy, the feeling of being totally alive and yet sheltered by life can only come about when all the chakras are opened to an equal extent and their frequencies are vibrating on the highest plane they can achieve.

An attitude of unconditional acceptance requires a great deal of honesty and courage. Honesty in this context means the readiness to see ourselves with all our weaknesses and negative characteristics, and not the way we would like to imagine ourselves. Courage is the readiness to accept what we see. It is the willingness to say "yes" to everything, without exception.

In our lives we have taken on our parents' judgement of us in order to retain their love, we have suppressed certain emotions and wishes in order to live up to the expectations of society, a group or an ideal. Giving all this up means relying solely on ourselves and losing the love and recognition of those around us, as we mistakenly believe. Yet it is only the act of rejecting, of negation, that lets the energies in us assume negative forms of expression. The repressed emotions only turn "bad" because we reject them instead of facing them with love and understanding. The more forcefully they are rejected, the more bad and torturous they become, until maybe at some point we liberate them with our love.

Behind every emotion there is, lastly, the yearning to regain the original, paradisiacal condition of unity. But as soon as we conform to the world's predominant way of viewing things and accept as real only the outer level of reality, as perceived physical senses and the rational mind, this wish for oneness, for unity with all of life, turns into a desire to possess. Our desire to own or possess a person, a position, love and recognition as well as material goods, however, is always disappointed anew, or else does not provide us with durable fulfillment as expected. This can only be achieved through inner oneness.

Out of fear of new disappointment we hold back our energies - and our energy system is blocked. Energies moving up are distorted by the blockage and express themselves as negative emotions, which again we frequently try to hold back and suppress in order not to loose the affection of those around us.

We can interrupt this cycle of cause and effect by giving our emotions our undivided attention. At that very moment they will begin to change, for we finally recognize that they are merely energies, brought forth by the yearning for oneness and blocked in their original expression. They now become a power that will help us on our way towards wholeness.

A simple analogy may illustrate this. If you are afraid of a person and reject him, you will never get to know his entire being. But if you give him your attention and let him feel your unconditional love, he will gradually open up to you. You will recognize that behind his negative behavior, which you condemned, lies nothing but a disappointed yearning for fulfillment. Your understanding will help him to start on the path towards genuine fulfillment. In this analogy your emotions undergo the same process this person does.

This attitude of unbiased acceptance corresponds to the attitude of our Higher Self. By consciously adopting it we open ourselves to the vibrational plane of the inner guide within us and assign it the task of leading us to complete health and wholeness.

The Higher Self is that part of our soul which connects us to the Divine Being. It is not limited by time and space. Therefore it always has access to the entire store of knowledge regarding all life in the universe as well as our own lives. If we entrust ourselves to its guidance it will lead us to inner unity by the straightest and most direct way, and the blockages within our energy system will be resolved as the most gentle way conceivable.

If we understand these principles, we will be able to apply the therapies described in this book with maximum effect. Always let the feelings that come up during therapy flow, even if they appear unpleasant or negative. In this case give them your unbiased attention and your love, and consign them to the healing power of your Higher Self.

There are forms of meditation that can help you practise such an attitude of acceptance, that will help you dissolve your blockages, and permit the self-healing powers of your Higher Self to do their job. One of these meditation techniques, which we can recommend from personal experience, is Transcendental Meditation, called TM for short. Utilizing the most direct approach, it leads one's consciousness without any effort or concentration towards the experience of pure being. This process is accompanied by an increasing serenity in which the blocked energies are freed by themselves. The thoughts and emotions being liberated are not rejected, but are replaced instead by a feeling of increasing relaxation and joy. This form of meditation is an effective tool, which, if used properly, will activate your chakras in a harmonious manner, cleanse your energy system of blockages, and help you realize your entire mental and spiritual potential. TM can only be learned through a qualified teacher, however. Other types of meditation can also be of help on your way. But be sure that thoughts and feelings are not judged or rejected in the form of meditation you choose, but are integrated as part of the necessary cleansing process instead. Even in the most effective and natural forms of meditation you may start to judge what you experience, simply out of habit, or you may also want to suppress unpleasant experiences accompanying the dissolution of blockages. If this happens, your neutrality will be impaired and the effectiveness of the meditation may suffer. A properly trained teacher can help you to regain the correct attitude.

As soon as you have learned to love and accept yourself completely, you radiate these vibrations out through your aura and attract corresponding experiences from the outer world. This means that you really gain the love and recognition through others which you had been afraid of losing. They, in turn, begin to appreciate you for the way you are and may also admire you for the courage to be yourself. Genuine love and unity become possible only under these conditions.

We would like to mention one last point pertaining to the theme of this chapter. On your way to holistic development, you may experience phases in which your chakras will be relatively open without your having removed all the blockages. You will then be very receptive for energies entering your aura but will not be able to radiate the kind of vibrations that only attract constructive energies, nor will you be able to neutralize negative vibrations in your environment.

If in this state you should find yourself in a tense atmosphere dominated by vibrations of dissatisfaction, hostility or aggression, your chakras may be burdened with negative energies, or may contract in order to protect themselves. In both cases the result will be an insufficient supply of positive life energy.

Whenever two people's energy fields touch or overlap, a direct exchange and a mutual influencing of energies occurs. Unconsciously we perceive the energy level of the other person, whether we want to or not. When we spontaneously like or dislike someone the primary reason has to do with the nature of the energy vibrations we feel in his or her aura. If we sense fear, dissatisfaction or anger, these vibrations will not only influence our image of the person, but also our own energy system. When you feel tense or uncomfortable in someone's presence for no apparent reason, or perhaps even get the feeling that everything inside you is contracting, the cause for this will be the vibrations that person's aura radiates. On the other hand, if you discern joy, love and serenity in someone's aura, you will feel especially well in that person's presence without either of you having said a word.

The collective aura of a group of people gathered together for a common purpose can develop such a powerful influence that every member of the group is swept away by it - we need only recall the common feeling that develops in audiences at sports events. And when a group of people gathers for prayer or meditation, the individual member may be raised to levels of consciousness much higher than those normally possible.

Places have their own aura, too, as matter is also capable of storing vibrations. This occurs to an especially high degree in enclosed areas.
We believe that it is particularly important to understand these correlations as they apply to our contact with small children. The young human being's energy system is still perfectly receptive for all kinds of energy vibrations. It is especially sensitive to all loving thoughts and feelings of joy, but also for tension, dispute and aggressiveness in its surroundings. The bodily presence of a parent or other trusted adult therefore represents valuable protection when the child is exposed to a multitude of strange vibrations, for instance while shopping. The adult's aura will act as a

buffer shielding the child from harmful vibrations. This is another reason why it is preferable to carry children instead of having them lie in a baby carriage.

As adults we can do a great deal to help our own chakras as well as those of our children to stay relaxed and open. Although we fundamentally attract the vibrations and situations that correspond to our own energy radiation, we do have a certain leeway in determining the exterior circumstances of our life, too. We can, for instance, take part in activities that will generate an atmosphere of love and joy. We can go to places that radiate positive, uplifting energy, and we can transform our own home into such a place. Pleasant colors, flowers, fragrances and relaxing music can do a lot to help bring about a harmonious, affirmative atmosphere. By determining which television programs, conversations and activities we partake of in our home, we can create an atmosphere in which the energy system of every person present is able to relax and regenerate.

There is a lot you can do for your inner sphere, too, especially to protect yourself from unwanted influences from your environment. We therefore recommend you to pay special attention to the opening of your heart chakra when undergoing character therapy, as love radiated away from you will be able to neutralize or transform all negative vibrations. The capability of unfolding your love along with other aspects represents a special challenge.

Additionally, the development of your heart chakra will make you increasingly aware and appreciative of the positive sides of others, automatically letting only these vibrations enter you. By your appreciation these qualities will simultaneously be strengthened and vitalized in the other person. Every encounter can become a gain for each of the persons involved.

Actively radiating vibrations will be a good protection in all cases. As soon as you have learned to accept yourself as you are and to openly radiate your energies, negative vibrations from your environment will no longer be able to penetrate your aura. When you are perfectly serene and relaxed within yourself, exterior tension will not be able to resonate within, nor will it be able to take hold of you or influence you negatively. We are, of course, aware of the fact that these capabilities require a fairly advanced stage of development. We therefore want to mention a few additional, simple methods you may wish to use in order to protect yourself from unwanted influence or to defend yourself against negative energies.

If, in a given situation you want to protect yourself or increase your own influence, imagine yourself drawing light into your body through your crown chakra and, again using your imagination, see yourself radiating it through your solar plexus chakra and thereby enclosing your body in a protective wrapping of light which illuminates and dissolves all negative influences. Imagine the light radiating away from your solar plexus chakra as strong as a waterfall, sweeping away all of those negative vibrations.

Ethereal oils are also an effective form of protection, and for this purpose you should apply them directly to the chakras. They will fill your aura with pure radiation and neutralize tensions and disharmonious influences entering your aura from the outside.

If you carry a rock crystal on your person it will intensify the quality of the light of your aura and its protective sheathe. The effect of rock crystals and ethereal oils augment each other very well.

Undergarments of silk also provide protection, and are particularly recommended for infants and toddlers. If at one time or another you find yourself very upset by sudden fright, shock or anger, we would like to recommend another effective method that will let you rid yourself of accumulated energy immediately. Stand with your feet slightly apart and tense up your muscles as hard as you can for several seconds. If you are alone, scream as loudly as possible, and if not, just empty your lungs of air in one blast. Repeat this exercise until you feel better. It will loosen the blockages caused by the fact that your energy system was unable to cope with the sudden experience. If it feels good, you may wish to stretch your body extensively, as if you had just awoken from a deep, relaxing sleep. It is interesting to note that in some people the phenomenon of muscle tension will occur spontaneously during meditation, and then in those parts of their bodies in which they are trying to loosen blockages. This is a clear indication of the usefulness and effectiveness of this exercise.

How to Determine Which Chakras Are Blocked

As this book provides a number of methods for the harmonization and opening of your chakras, you will want to know whether your chakras are blocked or out of balance and if so, which ones. Without this specific information you could apply all the therapeutic methods described here, simply to harmonize the chakras - a holistic method of treatment to be strongly recommended, anyway. However, if you are in a position to realize that two chakras need to be treated more than the others, you will be able to give them the required attention accordingly.

Becoming aware of the state of your chakras also provides you with a grand opportunity to get to know yourself better. Remember, however, you are the person who counts in this process, not the others. Of course, you can tell other people about what you're experiencing, but the idea is not to "convert" anyone, but rather to get to know and liberate ourselves, and then, if possible, to lovingly lead the other person on the same road to self-recognition.

There are several different methods of diagnosing the state of the chakras. If you choose to take advantage of only one, it may be all you need to effectively diagnose the chakra systems in yourself and others.

1. Along with the description of each chakra, this book provides you with knowledge of the characteristics by which you can determine which of your chakras are in a harmonious state and which are out of harmony or not functioning properly. These criteria will enable anyone to quickly determine his or her problem areas. In presenting this information we have purposely depicted the effects of chakra dysfunction to the point of exaggeration, thus hoping to make it easier to recognize certain tendencies. While reading these passages you should keep in mind that not everyone will be affected in the same way. Yet certain parts of the text may make a deep impression, or even make you feel you are being attacked. This is certainly not our intention. All we want to do is help you to see yourself clearly and to recognize yourself, where applicable. If some of the descriptions seem to apply to you, they should make you stop and think. Please do not see such descriptions as accusations. It is not our intention to hurt you, but simply to assist you in gaining awareness, but it must be remembered that self-recognition is not always pleasant. However, our darker sides want to be illuminated, because it is the only

way they can be liberated, and this path towards self-knowledge is definitely worth following. Apart from which, it entails a number of methods for harmonizing and treating the chakras yourself.

2. Another method of analysing our chakras consists of closely observing which chakras react noticeably in situations of unusual stress or shock. Perhaps you always notice the same complaints in yourself when certain difficult situations occur. If, for instance, the root chakra is not functioning sufficiently, you may have the feeling that you are loosing your footing or that the rug is being pulled from under your feet when you are subjected to heavy pressure, or you might even suffer from diarrhea. On the other hand, if your root chakra is overfunctioning, you may work yourself up into anger or aggression in similar situations. Underfunctioning of the second chakra for its part will cause a blockage of your feelings when you experience anxiety, while a hyperfunction will probably make you break out into tears or let you react with an uncontrollable show of feelings. To turn to the third chakra, impaired functioning here will let you feel powerless when under pressure can manifest in the form of a queasy feeling in your stomach or helpless nervousness, while overfunctioning will be marked by nervous irritability and the attempt to control a given situation through hyperactivity. When a situation causes you to feel that your heart has "skipped a beat", the functioning of your heart chakra is most likely impaired. If, on the other hand, your pulse races in stress situations, the reason may be a general dysfunction of the heart chakra. Hypoactivity of the throat chakra gives you a "lump" in the throat and a generally constricted feeling, you begin to stutter or your head may begin to quiver starting out at the neck, while hyperactivity may make you try to salvage the situation with a torrent of unconsidered words. The inability to think clearly under conditions of stress or shock indicates, finally, an underfunctioning of the inner eye chakra, while overfunctioning of the same often manifests itself in the form of headaches.

Reactions such as these always occur at weakened points in our energy system. Close observation may serve to open our eyes.

3. We can also employ the appearance of the body and body language to determine which chakras are blocked. Our bodies are merely exemplary mirror images of our subtle energy structures. Whenever abnormal bodily characteristics manifest themselves, be it in the form of curvatures, swellings, tenseness, weakness etc., we can determine the relationship with the chakra in question depending on the part of the body where they occur. We all know the differences in appearances, that enable us to create a mental picture of someone without too much difficulty. Our idea

of someone can often be transferred to the chakra situation and thus provide us with useful information. We all come across people who have apparently drawn all their energy into the upper part of the body, to the detriment of the lower part, which is correspondingly weak in configuration. In other people we may find the exact opposite, while yet others again seem to consist entirely of weakness or strength. With this in mind, take a good, conscious look at yourself in a mirror or in photographs. The human voice is often an important indicator of the state of a person's throat chakra.

If, in addition to this, you take symptoms of chronic and acute conditions into consideration, you will soon know which chakras are beset by deficiencies and can then proceed to treat them accordingly.

The chapters on the individual chakras contain all the details regarding the connection between the chakras, the organs and areas of the body. Using this information, you can determine where the dysfunctions are localized and employ the therapy of your choice to correct them.

4. As a fourth possibility we would like to mention a special method of testing that many therapists and lay practitioners use to the exclusion of all others. It is known as the "kinesiological test"* and was developed as part of the "Touch for Health" method. If you try it out on yourself, you will need someone to help you.

The test is carried out as follows. Place your right hand on a chakra and at the same time extend your left arm away from your body at a right angle. The other person, who is testing you, now gives the command "hold on", and while you try to maintain your arm in the original position, your partner tries to push it down by applying pressure in the area of the wrist. If the chakra is in harmony and functioning smoothly, the extended arm will offer clearly felt, strong resistance. If, however, the chakra being tested is blocked, this will be easily determined by its lack of resistance. Your partner will be able to depress it with a minimum of effort.

Using this method we test all the chakras from the root center up to the crown center, thus gaining a clear picture of the energetic condition of each chakra. The arm test will always indicate disturbances in a given chakra if the arm reacts weakly. We can repeat the test at a later time to determine changes that may have taken place. If a chakra system is free of disturbances, the arm-test score will be "strong" in all seven instances

*»Dein Körper lügt nicht« * , Dr. John Diamond, Verlag für angewandte Kinesiologie, Freiburg, 1983

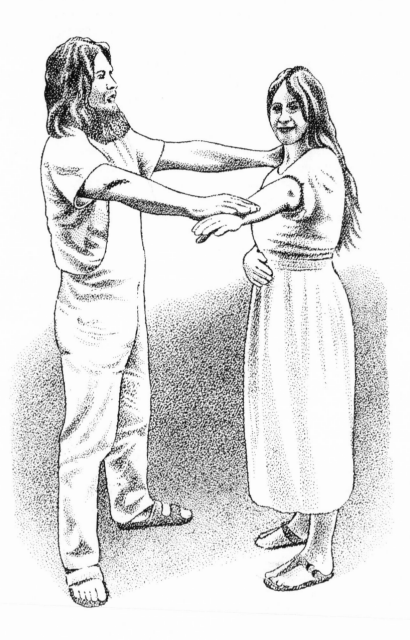

Kinesiological muscle test

and the attempt to depress the arm will be met with clearly felt resistance in every case. It is advisable to rest between testing the individual chakras to avoid tiring the arm.

Measurements with a specially constructed kinesiometer have shown that a "strong" rating is equal to about 44 lbs. of downward pressure, whereas about 18 lbs. of pressure will usually suffice to push the arm down. An important factor here is, of course, the individual physique. But regardless of the physical characteristics or bodily strength of the person being tested, both partners will be able to clearly differentiate between "strong" and "weak" arm control.

A variation of the test consists of pressing together thumb and forefinger of the right hand and covering the chakra to be tested with the left hand. Our test partner now attempts to pull thumb and forefinger apart once the command is given. If this proves to be difficult, the chakra in question is sound, but if resistance is weak, the chakra is disturbed in some way and requires attention.

On several occasions we have met people who apply this test to themselves. While mentally focussing on a given chakra, they press thumb and forefinger of one hand together and attempt to pull them apart with the other hand. This version of the test also clearly shows which chakras are not functioning properly. If the thumb and forefinger can be pulled apart easily, the condition is considered "weak" and that particular chakra is disturbed. If the thumb and forefinger remain closed, the chakra's state is "strong" and healthy. Of course, we need a certain amount of practise for these kinesiological tests in order to arrive at reliable results. The methods are excellent, however, and will reliably show which chakras need harmonizing work.

5. We call a further method for appraising the state of the chakras "looking within". For many people this is the simplest and quickest way of establishing contact with their energy system.

We enter into a meditative state of stillness for a few minutes and then try to gain an idea of the state of each individual chakra with our "inner eyes". Here again we systematically move through the chakras one by one, starting at the bottom. In doing this, many people can tell by changes in color what condition their chakras are in. (The meanings of the various colors are included in the detailed descriptions of the individual chakras. Any deviations from these colors should be considered as a signal.) Some people see shapes while doing this. If this is the case, watch to see if the shapes are round and harmoniously balanced, or if they show indentations or other changes. Still others recognize the state of their chakras by their size and glow. Frequently a combination of these various manifestations will be perceived. All these methods and criteria of assessing the chakras require a certain amount of self-experience and need to be practised repeatedly in order to produce reliable and understandable results.

6. Increasing numbers of people are developing the capability of assessing their energy situation by "feeling" around their subtle bodies with their hands. This is often referred to as "tactile clairvoyance." This method enables you to feel a certain resistance when you come upon the energy mantle of your own ethereal body, where the chakras are located, or that of another person. This resistance has the feeling of movements made under water. You may detect a certain unevenness, as well as holes and bumps. We can practise this by approaching our own body or that of another person or animals and plants slowly with our hands while trying to determine the changes that take place. Here, too, repeated practise is essential if clear results are to be obtained. We recommend attending a workshop in which this can be learned.

7. The most direct way of assessing the chakras is by employing the ability to see auras, but very few people possess this gift. With it, the "seer" has direct access to the energetic situation and processes taking place in himself and other people. Seeing the chakras makes it possible to recognize and evaluate the spiritual, psychic and physical relationships taking place. If you are blessed with these medial capabilities it will be very important that you interpret what you see properly, and this requires a great deal of training, experience and the ability to observe properly. A lot can be learned from the literature on this subject as well as through seminars.

Should you be uncertain of whether or not you have this talent, you can test yourself in the following manner: sit down in a completely light-proof room. (it doesn't matter what kind of enclosed space this is; Bodo, for example, conducted his first experiments in an air raid shelter - all that counts is that no light enters whatsoever.) Begin by spending several minutes in silence. As initial objects to be tested a few rock crystal points set up close to you or held in your hands will suffice. If you are capable of perceiving a certain subtle energy radiation emanating from the crystal points, especially when they are moved from side to side, you have a tendency towards visual clairvoyance. If you experience no immediate results, do not give up right away; in some cases this ability, too, needs to trained in order to manifest itself. While testing yourself remember not to attempt to force or strain yourself but to effortlessly let things happen. If you wish to see a person's energy body, it is advisable to have him or her sit or stand in front of a dark backdrop, if possible. From a distance of several yards you then look slightly above or beside the person, for this is where the ring of energy will be, the aura. Best results are achieved in a meditative state. Take your time. Presumably the first thing you will perceive will be the ethereal body surrounding the physical body like a glowing sheath of energy. Given the necessary practise you will be able to discern the colors and shapes of the astral body. Do not expect to see a static, motionless form of colors as the subtle energies are of a shimmering, semitransparent nature and in constant motion. Basically one can say that harmonious shapes and colors within these energy structures indicate a harmonious person, whereas muddled colors and unbalanced shapes indicate the person's problem areas.

If you wish to try to perceive your own aura, try out this method in front of a full-length mirror. Most people find it easier at the beginning to look for the energy radiation given off by someone else.

Additionally, there are special aura glasses available having dark-violet lenses and light-proofing all around. These glasses should be considered as supporting implements, and while they do not automatically provide every user access to the subtle planes, they really can assist us in our initial efforts. We have had very good experience with them, especially out-of-doors.

Today we also find that more and more people are capable of assessing and evaluating the chakras and the energy body of a given person over a distance of hundreds of miles. As a rule this is done using a photograph of the person seeking advice, or via the telephone. A lot of people do not find such methods very credible, but we have witnessed them a number of times and have frequently been involved ourselves.

If you have a problem accepting such extraordinary phenomena, please consider what radio and television are capable of today. In their case, too, words and pictures are invisibly transmitted over great distances. Practically all the advances that have been made in technology also exist as natural phenomena, including the wireless transmission of information.

You are free to reject certain methods and possibilities if they do not seem plausible to you. We have, after all, already listed a number of other methods for the evaluation of the chakras.

8. Another way of recognizing someone's chakra functions lies in the medial capability to feel in one's own chakras whatever the person seeking advice is experiencing and feeling. In order to do this, the therapist tunes in to the patient's energy body. We know several therapists who employ this method to arrive at definite diagnoses, but many of them feel like the person seeking help afterwards. We therefore feel that this

should is not a totally advisable method.

9.) In a number of traditional Asian texts, various characteristics for the dominant function of the chakras are named. In this context the analysis of our sleeping habits is of special interest.

If a person lives primarily through the first chakra, a greater need for sleep ranging from 10 to 12 hours will manifest itself, and the preferred sleeping position will be on the stomach. People requiring approximately 8 - 10 hours of sleep, which they spend in a prenatal position, live primarily through their second chakra. Those of us leading their lives mostly through the third chakra prefer sleeping on their backs and require 7 - 8 hours of sleep. A person whose fourth chakra is predominantly developed will usually rest on the left side and only needs 5 - 6 hours of sleep per night. If the fifth chakra is open and predominant, 4 - 5 hours of sleep are required each night, spent resting on the right and left side alternately. If the sixth chakra is opened, active and predominant, the person will only spend about 4 hours between sleep and waking sleep. Waking sleep is a state in which inner consciousness is maintained while the body sleeps. It is the type of rest to be expected when the seventh chakra is open and ruling. The totally enlightened person no longer sleeps in the usual sense, but simply provides the body periods of rest.

These characteristics represent an additional way for us to evaluate the functioning of our chakras.

Beside the methods described here, a number of technical developments stemming from the area of borderline science are available to us. These include pendulums and divining rods as well as Kirlian photography, which are used by some therapists for chakra analysis. Among the divining rods, the so-called pendulum rod, also referred to as a "Biotensor"*, is especially suitable. Employing this instrument makes it relatively easy to define the state the chakras are in, which also holds true for a pendulum. A stable chakra will cause it to swing in larger circles, while a disturbed chakra will result in smaller circles or may even bring the pendulum or rod to a standstill. Of course practise is required in this area, too, in order to enable us to clearly differentiate results.

Kirlian photography is a special technical process by which energetic radiation, given off for instance by parts of the body, is registered photographically and depicted in color. A great deal of attention is

* Described in *Das große Biotensor Praxis-Buch*, Dr. Josef Oberbach, Verlag Deutsche Bioplasma Forschung, Munich, 1983

currently being given to the energetic "terminal point diagnosis" developed by the nonmedical practitioner Peter Mandel on the basis of Kirlian photography.* A large number of medical professionals and nonmedical practitioners are already working with this bio-energetic method of diagnosis.

In Japan, highly refined electronic systems are being employed in order to reach diagnoses at the subtle level, but as we are more interested in making use of the ways and means nature has provided us with, we limit ourselves here to a brief mention of these technical devices.

If, finally, you decide to employ only one of the methods of chakra evaluation described here, it may be all you need. It is often better to master one skill completely, than to dabble in several at once. We therefore wish you successful implementation of the knowledge contained in these pages.

---

*) *Energy Emission Analysis,* Peter Mandel, Synthesis Verlag, Wessobrunn, Germany

Sexuality and the Chakras

Human sexuality is a means of expression and mirrors the eternal act of creation constantly taking place on all levels of life throughout the universe. When Oneness became Plurality at the moment of creation, formless being initially divided itself into two fundamental forms of energy - a fertile male force and a receptive female force. Thousands of years ago the Chinese named these primordial forces Yin and Yang. The interaction of these energies brings forth all Creation. The female Yin is unceasingly fertilized by the male seed of Yang and produces all of life's myriad forms.

At the physical human level this interaction of forces manifests itself as sexuality. Through it the human being is connected with the eternal act of the creation of life in its entirety, and the ecstasy he or she may experience is a reflection of the bliss of creation.

Within the entire universe the forces of Yin and Yang manifest themselves as polarity. In order to exist, everything has its opposite or counterpoint. Every point depends on its counterpoint in order to exist, and if one aspect of this polarity ceases to be, its opposite no longer exists either. This fundamental rule can be applied to everything. We can exhale only if we inhale, and if the one ceases, so does the other. The internal brings about the external, day brings about night, light brings about shadow, birth leads to death, woman leads to man, etc., whereby the two given polarities are always interchangeable. In order to be complete, every point must have its counterpoint.

Yin and Yang clearly symbolize the rhythmic movement of all life. Yin represents the female, extending, emotional, passive and unconscious part of the whole, whereas Yang stands for the male, contracting, active and conscious side. This, however, in no way represents a value judgement in the sense of one or the other possessing more worth.

The existing balance of the universe around us is the result of the interactions between the polarity pairs (points and counterpoints). Since everything in the universe is in continuous movement, Yin and Yang, too, each exist latently in their respective counterpoints. This is symbolized by the white dot in the dark Yin shape and the black dot in the white Yang shape. Each of the two poles already contains the seed of its counterpoint, and it is only a matter of time until one polarity transforms into the other. At some levels, such as that of atoms, this transformation occurs within a split second, whereas the polarity change between the male and female

UNITY

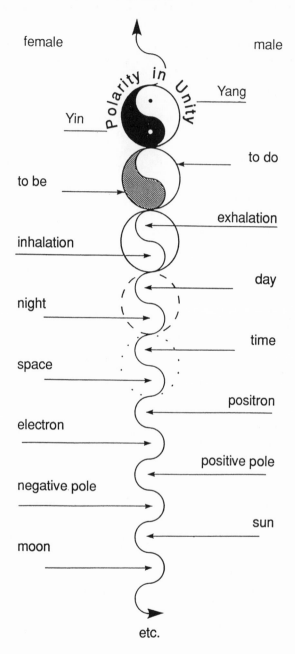

female   male

Polarity in Unity

Yin   Yang

to be   to do

inhalation   exhalation

night   day

space   time

electron   positron

negative pole   positive pole

moon   sun

etc.

principles at the human level always requires separate incarnations. Day and nicht only need an average of twelve hours for such a transformation, while inhaling and exhaling only take a few seconds.

All things come and go, are in a state of continuous movement and transformation due to the interaction of these two basic forms of energy in the universe, but it is only by the completion of both cycles that complete Oneness is achieved.

Love and sexuality are based on the same principle. Two poles push to melt into one, they attract one another like the poles of a magnet, and when the two opposite energies finally unite, they interchange.

Men and women are poled oppositely in all their basic characteristics, including the energetic level. Where men are poled positively, women are poled negatively, and vice versa. As we have already explained in the previous chapter, this phenomenon also applies to the direction in which the individual chakras rotate. (In cases of homosexuality, for instance, the energetic poling is contrary to the rule.) Consequently, there is attraction and fulfillment between the sexes on all the levels represented by the chakras, and this can bring about total and profound Oneness. In order for this to occur, the chakras have to be clear of all blockages. During sexual union the flow of energy along the main channel (*sushumna*) is extremely stimulated and intensified. The flow of energy in the second chakra increases enormously, and this abundance of energy will charge all the other chakras if the chakra system is not blocked. The sexual energy, representing a certain form of *prana*, is hereby transformed into the frequencies of the other chakras. Starting from the chakras, it radiates out through the nadis into the physical body and the energy bodies, charging them with heightened vital energy. At the climax of this union a tremendous energetic discharge in all seven chakras is achieved in both partners, and a fusion takes place on all levels represented by the chakras. Both partners are revitalized down to the depths of their being, and at the same time feel totally relaxed. The profound love and closeness they experience by far transcends any personal desire to possess. The relationship experiences a form of fulfillment totally independent of all external factors.

Such a fulfilling sexual union can only be attained in these dimensions, however, if the partners relate completely with each other and free themselves of all fears that might hinder the free flow within their energy systems. If only one chakra is blocked in one of the partners, the union cannot be experienced in this perfection. Moreover, the blocked chakra creates a disturbance within the energy flow of the corresponding chakra of the partner.

Most people experience sexuality only via the second chakra. In addition, the energy of the root chakra plays a dominant role in the male sex as a physical driving force. If sexuality remains limited to the lower chakras, it becomes a rather unilateral experience which tends to leave both partners weakened and dissatisfied, inclined to separate quickly and go back to being alone again. This is comparable to strumming merely one or two strings of a musical instrument; the entire spectrum of sounds it is capable of will never ring out. In fact, from an energetic point of view a great deal of energy is exhausted by such sexual practice, as energies are drained from other chakras and transformed into sexual energy in order to stream out through the second chakra. In this way, the energies are prevented from taking their natural way to the top, flowing simultaneously into all seven chakras and charging them with additional vital force.

The most natural way to dissolve the blockages which impair complete sexual union at all levels is an exchange of the heart chakra's energies. If both partners radiate the love from their heart freely and without fear, their own energy system as well as that of the other person will harmonize increasingly. Fear and anxiety blockages will dissolve and an exchange

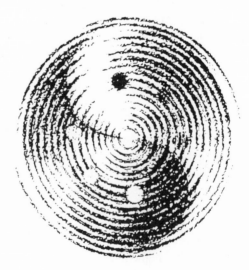

The interplay of polarities

becomes possible at the levels of all seven chakras. This is the reason why we experience far greater fulfillment in sexual union when, in addition to mutual physical attraction, partners are united in a profound state of love. In this case, higher energy frequencies are activated, lifting sexuality beyond the purely physical and letting it evolve into spiritual union.

This is the art of Tantra, which has been taught and practiced for thousands of years. In applying it, the orgasmic experience becomes one of far greater, forceful proportions than is generally considered possible. Experiencing this really does lead us into the realm of another dimension of sensation and perception. We suddenly become aware that our sexual energies are not locked up in our genitals, but are present in every single cell of our body, as well as in the interaction of female and male forces in all the manifestations of creation. Perfect union with a beloved partner lets us experience inner oneness with the pulsating life of the universe. At the moment of climax, when duality is briefly transcended, we experience unity with the absolute, formless Being which is the firm basis and objective of the interaction of polarity.

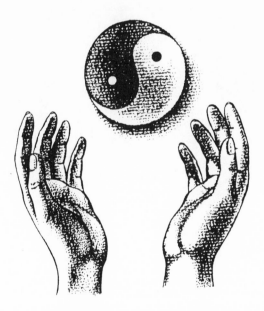

The game of life: unity and duality

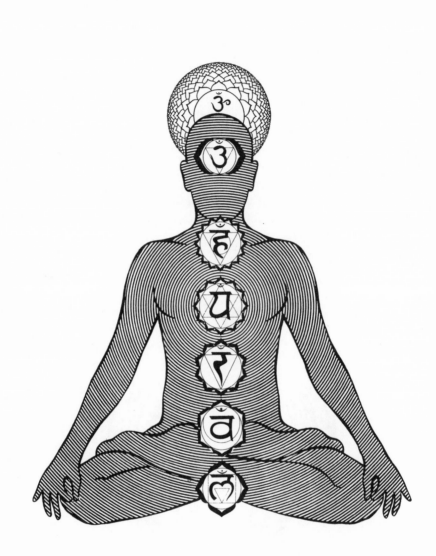

The First Chakra

Muladhara Chakra,
also called the Root Center,
the Base Chakra or the Coccyx Center

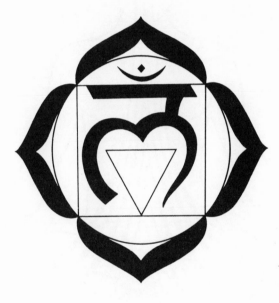

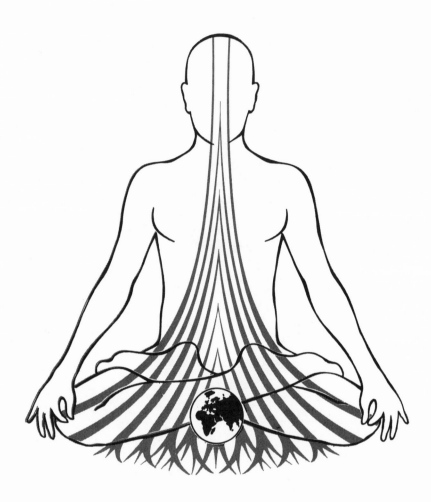

The first chakra is located between the anus and the genitals. It is connected with the coccyx and opens downward.

The First Chakra and Its Associated Characteristics

Color: An active first chakra shines in a fiery red

Associated element: Earth

Sense: Smell

Symbols: 4-petaled lotus

Basic principle: Physical will of being (in contrast to the spiritual will of being in the seventh chakra)

Associated parts of the body: All solid parts like the spinal column, bones, teeth, and nails. Anus, rectum, colon, prostate gland. Blood and the building of cells.

Associated glands: Suprarenal glands.
The suprarenal glands produce adrenaline and noradrenaline, which have the function of adapting the blood circulation to our needs by regulating blood distribution. In this way our body is able to immediately react to differing demands. Moreover, the suprarenal glands have a dominating influence upon the balance of temperature in our body.

Associated astrological signs and planets:
Aries/Mars: New beginning, primordial life energy, power to achieve, aggressiveness.
Taurus: Closeness to earth, stability, possession, sensual pleasure.
Scorpio/Pluto: Unconscious attachment, sexual power, transformation and renewal.
Capricorn/Saturn: Structure and stability.

The *Ayurvedic teachings* also assign the sun, as the primordial source of all life, to the root chakra.

Purpose and function of the first chakra

The root chakra connects us with the physical world. It transfers cosmic energies to the physical and earthly level and lets earthly energy stream into our subtle system.

Here we enter into contact with the "spirit of Mother Earth" and are able to experience her elemental force, her love and patience. Man's basic individual and global needs for life and survival on this planet belong to the sphere of influence of the first chakra.

Those who succeed in opening it will fully accept life on earth, they will say "yes" to their physical existence and will be prepared to live and act in harmony with the earthly forces and learn from them.

As the root chakra is assigned to the earthly element, its color is red - the red of the energy and activity welling up from the inner core of our planet. It gives us earthly stability and the "solid ground" upon which we can construct our lives. At the same time, it provides us with the necessary energy for creative self-expression. Moreover, it lends us the power to achieve and consistency.

Building up an existence, finding material security and securing the survival of the species by founding a family belong to the sphere of this first chakra, along with sexuality as a physical function and a means of begetting children.

The root chakra forms the vital foundation for all the higher chakras and is the source of the life force. Here we are in touch with the inexhaustible reservoir of *kundalini* energy. *Sushumna*, *ida* and *pingala*, the three main energy channels of the human body, also begin in this chakra. As the heart in the body, so the root chakra forms the center of our system of subtle energy cycles. Moreover, it is the true seat of the collective unconscious. It is through this chakra that the stored knowledge of the collective unconscious becomes accessible. In order to maintain our inner balance, the root chakra should always function in harmony with the seventh chakra.

Harmonious functioning

If your root chakra is open and working harmoniously, you will experience a deep, personal relationship with Earth and the life forms it nurtures. Your life energy will be intact, you will be rooted in life and yourself, and your life is characterized by satisfaction, stability and inner strength. You feel embedded in natural life cycles, in the alternation of rest and activity, death and renewed birth; your actions are guided by the desire to be creatively active in shaping life on your mother planet, always in accordance with the generating force of Earth and all life in nature. It will be easy for you to achieve your goals in this world. Your life is sustained by an unshakable primordial trust. Your perceive the earth as a secure place which provides you with everything you need: care, food, shelter and security. Trustingly you open yourself to life on earth and accept everything it holds in store for you with gratitude.

Disharmonious functioning

If your root chakra malfunctions or becomes unbalanced, your thoughts and actions primarily revolve around material possessions and security, or sensual indulgences and thrills, such as good food, alcohol, sex, etc. You want to make whatever you desire your own without considering the consequences. At the same time, you find it rather difficult to give or take freely. You have a marked tendency to maintain security and distance. On the physical plane, the inability to let go and the desire to maintain possession often manifest themselves as constipation and overweight.

Your actions revolve primarily around satisfying your own personal needs and you unconsciously overlook or ignore the needs of others as well as those of your own body for healthy, moderate nourishment, sufficient rest and a balanced and harmonious way of life.

In the extreme, you adhere to certain attitudes and lusts of which you cannot rid yourself. If your fixations are challenged by people or situations, you become easily irritated or upset, sometimes even furious or aggressive. Violent enforcement of your will and principles is another manifestation of a disturbed root chakra.

In the final analysis, rage, anger and violence are only defense mechanisms which indicate a lack of primordial trust. Behind this there is always a fear of losing something which provides you with security and a feeling of well-being, or of not gaining it in the first place.

For you the earth is a place to be dominated and exploited under the pretext of securing the survival of mankind. Therefore the present-day exploitation of natural resources and the destruction of the earth's natural balance are symptomatic of the disrupted functioning of the root chakra in the majority of the world's population.

Insufficient functioning

If your root chakra is blocked or closed, your physical constitution tends to be weak and you lack physical and emotional stamina. A lot of things in life worry you and you are only too familiar with feelings of uncertainty. You may have the feeling that you have lost your footing or that you are floating in the air or are "not all there". It may be difficult for you to meet the demands of everyday life and you frequently lack stability and the power to achieve. All too often, life on this earth is a burden instead of a pleasure and most of the time you long for an easier, more pleasant and less strenuous way of life.

If your higher chakras have been developed to the detriment of the lower ones, the feeling that you don't really belong on the earth may indicate a state of insufficiency in your root chakra. If your sacral chakra and the solar plexus chakra are also blocked, anorexia may set in as you absorb hardly any elemental life force through your root chakra, and is a symptom of your wish to flee. However, you will continue to be faced with the problems of earthly life until you learn to accept them as milestones on your way to holistic development.

Possibilities for cleansing and activating the first chakra

Experiencing nature

The contemplation of a blood-red sun rising or setting, or of a radiant dawn or sunset, revives and harmonizes the root chakra and loosens the confined structures within its sphere.

In order to get in touch with the comforting, stabilizing and revitalizing energy of our planet through the first chakra, sit on the ground in the lotus position and consciously breathe in its fragrance.

If you are able to combine both these nature experiences, this will have an optimal holistic effect on your root chakra.

Sound Therapy

Music: The appropriate music to activate the root chakra should consist of monotonous, emphatic rhythms. The ancient music of many primitive tribes best expresses these rhythms. Their dances also serve the purpose of establishing contact with nature, with all her energy and life forms.

In order to harmonize the root chakra, you can utilize the sounds of nature. If you do not have access to them in their original settings, cassettes and records will also do.

Vowel: The vowel "u" (spoken as 'ooh') is assigned to the root chakra, and should be sung in the lower C. The "u" sound sets off a downward movement towards your roots. It leads you into the depths of your unconscious and vitalizes the original, earthly power of the first chakra.

Mantra: LAM

Color therapy

The first chakra is activated by a clear, bright shade of red. The red color warms and revitalizes and awakens the life force, vitality and courage. If this red is tinged with a shade of blue, it will help you permeate your vital drives with spiritual energy.

Gemstone therapy

Agate: The agate provides seriousness, firmness and equanimity. It helps dissolve negative emotions and protects the inner Self. It stimulates esteem for your own body and activates the reproductive organs. Agates with crystalline inclusions protect and shelter any form of life growing within you, be it physical or mental. They strengthen trust and help alleviate the pains of delivery.

Hematite: The hematite provides strength and energy. It has a revitalizing effect on the body and mobilizes hidden energies. Thus it helps us overcome states of weakness and supports convalescence following an illness. Moreover, it stimulates a healthy build-up of the blood and cells.

Blood jasper: The green-red blood jasper connects you with the elementary power and patient love of "Mother Earth". It teaches you selflessness and modesty, strengthens your blood and lends you vitality and stability, strength and patience. It cleanses and transforms the physical body and conveys a feeling of security within the natural life cycle, from which we draw inner strength and serenity.

Garnet: The garnet provides drive, willpower, self-confidence and success. It opens our eyes for the yet unknown, and supports clairvoyance. It stimulates the sexual drive and helps to change it into a transforming and revitalizing energy. On a physical level, it helps to heal diseases of the genitals and stimulates the blood circulation.

Red coral: The red coral lends vital and flowing energy. It has a stimulating influence and supports the production of blood cells. It provides stability and, at the same time, encourages flexibility, helping you to remain firmly rooted within your own Self while flowing along the stream of life.

Ruby: The ruby lends a vital and warm creative energy which leads to purification and transformation. It establishes a harmonic synthesis between physical and spiritual love, between sexuality and spirituality, thus opening us up for new forms of experience.

Aroma therapy

Cedar: The tangy fragrance of cedarwood oil connects you with the earthly forces and all forms of natural life. It helps build up energy and conveys serenity and a feeling of security in the lap of "Mother Earth".

Clove: Oil of clove helps dissolve dammed-up energies within the root chakra. It encourages the readiness to liberate yourself from old and restricting social patterns originating out of a need for protection and security, and helps you open yourself to new, fresh energies. Thus if you will tune to the message of its vibrations, it will lead you to transformation and renewal .

Forms of Yoga that work primarily through the first chakra

Hatha Yoga: Unfolding of awareness through cleansing and stimulation of the physical body by the means of certain bodily exercises or postures combined with breathing exercises.

Kundalini Yoga: Awakening of the so-called "snake power", which starts at the coccyx and rises parallel to the spinal column. As it rises it activates and vitalizes all other chakras. There are myriads of physical and spiritual exercises that will help you achieve this effect.

The Second Chakra

Svadhistana Chakra,
also called the Sacral Chakra
or the Cross Center

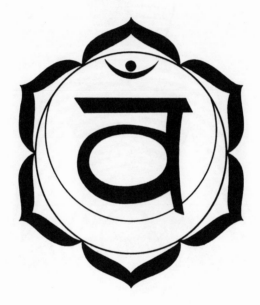

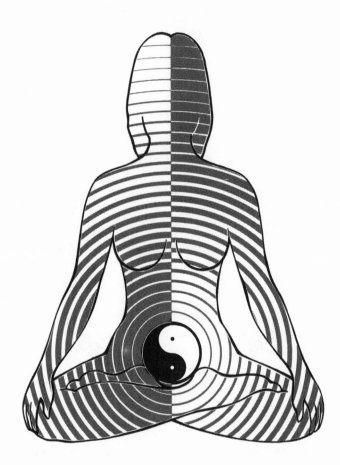

The second chakra is located above the genitals. It is connected with the sacrum (lat.: os sacrum) and opens towards the front.

The Second Chakra and its Associated Characteristics

Color: Orange

Associated element: Water

Sense: Taste

Symbols: 6-petalled lotus

Basic principle: Creative reproduction of being

Physical assignment: Pelvic girdle, reproductive organs, kidneys, bladder. All liquids such as blood, lymph, gastric juice, sperm.

Associated glands: Gonads - ovaries, prostate gland, testicles. The function of the gonads consists of manifesting the male and female sexual characteristics as well as the regulation of the female cycle.

Associated astrological signs and planets:
Cancer/Moon: Richness of feeling, receptiveness, fertility.
Libra/Venus: Attention to one's Self, relationships based on partnership. Sensuality, creativity.
Scorpio/Pluto: Sensual desire, transformation of personality through the giving up of one's own ego in sexual union.

Please note: Sometimes the second chakra is referred to as the spleen center. This, however, is an important secondary center which is closely related with the third chakra. This modification of the original chakra system originated in the negation of sexuality in some esoteric schools of thought, and later on various schools of though combined the aspects of differing systems. This is the reason why sexuality is often assigned to the spleen chakra of the root center.

Purpose and function
of the second chakra

The second chakra is the center of unfiltered primordial emotions, sexual energies and creativity. It is assigned to the element of water, the source of all biological life, and corresponds to the emotional sphere on the astrological plane.

Water fertilizes and continuously produces new life. Through the sacral chakra we participate in the fertilizing and receiving of energies which permeate the whole of nature. We see ourselves as parts of the everlasting process of creation which expresses itself in us as feeling and creativity.

The sacral chakra is often considered to be the real seat of Shakti, the "female" aspect of God in the form of creative energy. Its sphere of influence includes the male reproductive organs which carry within them the impulse to create new life, and in women the areas in which they receive creative impulses and generate new life, in the areas where the growing being is nourished, sheltered and provided with everything it needs for its development.

However, the water element also cleanses and purifies. It dissolves and washes away blockages that hinder its vital flow. On the physical plane, this is expressed by the decontaminating functions of the kidneys and bladder; on the spiritual level it manifests in the form of liberated, free-flowing feelings which make us willing to see life as something ever-primordial and new.

Our interpersonal relationships, especially those with the opposite sex, are influenced decisively by the functions of the second chakra. The manifold manifestations of Eros belong to its sphere, as well as the desire to renounce the limitations of the ego and experience greater wholeness in sexual union.

Harmonious functioning

The harmonious functioning of an open sacral chakra displays itself in the natural flow of life and feelings; you open yourself towards others, especially people of the opposite sex, and behave naturally. Sexual union with a beloved partner presents you with an opportunity to participate in the dance of creation performed by the male and female energies, thus helping you to experience an all-embracing sense of union with nature and gradually grow towards inner wholeness.

When the sacral chakra is functioning harmoniously, you feel the flow of creative life energy streaming through your body, soul and mind. By means of this stream you participate in the deep joy of creation and life continually fills you with awe and enthusiasm. Your feelings are genuine and undistorted, your actions are creative. They stimulate not only your own life but also the lives of others.

Disharmonious functioning

A malfunctioning of the sacral chakra often originates during puberty. The awakening sexual energies cause a state of uncertainty, and parents and educators are rarely capable of teaching young people how to handle these energies. Frequently, there has been a lack of tenderness and bodily contact stemming from early infancy. This may later lead to a negation and rejection of sexuality. As a consequence, the uninhibited expression of the creative potential of sexuality is lost and its energies can only be manifested in an inappropriate way, often through excessive sexual phantasies or suppressed desires which tend to erupt from time to time. It may also result in your using sex like a drug. Here, the creative potential of sexuality is not recognized or is misdirected. In both cases we find uncertainty and tensions regarding the other sex. Your sensuality is relatively coarse and you tend to force the satisfaction of your sexual desires into the foreground.

Or perhaps you simply live in constant yearning for a fulfilling sexual relationship, without being aware of the fact that the reason why you cannot achieve this lies within yourself.

With the loss of natural uninhibited and innocence in dealing with sexual energies you condemn the expression of these energies in Nature, and are no longer open for the interaction of the forces of Yin and Yang, nor can you feel a childlike amazement at the miracles of life.

Insufficient functioning

In most cases the cause of inadequate functioning of the sacral center can be traced back to childhood and infancy. Probably your parents held back their own sensuality and sexuality and you experienced a lack of sensual stimulation in the form of touches, caresses, tenderness and affection. As a consequence, you suppressed your feelings in this sphere and withdrew the antennas which receive sensual messages.

During puberty, you blocked off your developing sexual energies completely. The result of this "successful" suppression is a lack of self-esteem, emotional paralysis and sexual coldness. Life seems dreary to you, and you feel it is not really worth living.

Possibilities for cleansing and activating the second chakra

Experiencing nature

Moonlight and the contemplation or touching of clear water out-of-doors stimulate the second chakra. The moon, especially when it is full, brightens your feelings and makes you receptive for the messages of your soul as revealed through your imagination or dreams.

The quiet contemplation of in a clear natural body of water or immersement in it, or a few mouthfuls of water directly from a spring will help you cleanse and purify your soul and free it from emotional blockages and congestions, meaning that the life force within you can flow again unhindered.

If you are able to combine the contemplation of the moon with contact with water, the effect on the second chakra will be outstanding.

Sound therapy

Music: Any kind of "flowing" music which awakens a carefree joy in life is suitable for activating the second chakra. The flowing rhythms of folk and pair dances also belong to this category. Otherwise, you can use any kind of music which lets your emotions flow.

To calm down and harmonize the energies of the sacral chakra, you can listen to birdsong, the sound of running water or even the splashing melody of a small fountain, whether indoors or outdoors.

Vowel: The sacral chakra is activated by a closed »o«, like the »o« in the word »November«, and should be sung in D. The vowel »o« sets off a circular movement. At the end of the sound, when it approaches a »u«, it awakens emotional depth and leads to a state of circular unity, where Yin and Yang interact to form a harmonious whole.

In many languages the exclamation »oh!« expresses emotional amazement. Thus the ability to be astonished at the miracles of Creation is also revitalized by the vowel »o«.

Mantra: VAM.

Color therapy

A clear shade of orange activates the second chakra. The color orange supplies us with a stimulating, renewing energy and frees us from rigid emotional patterns. It encourages our self-esteem and increases the joy we get from sensual pleasures. According to Ayurveda, orange is the inner color of water.

Gemstone therapy

Carnelian: The carnelian brings you into contact with the beauty and creative energy of the earth. It helps you to live fully in the present and stimulates your concentration. It brings back your awe at the miracles of Creation, lets the life force flow anew and enlivens creative, expressive forces.

Moonstone: The moonstone opens you up to your own emotional richness. It connects you with the sensitive, receptive and dreamlike part of yourself and helps you to accept this side of yourself and integrate it into your personality. It takes away your fear of emotions and has a harmonizing effect on emotional balance.

On a physical level, it encourages the cleansing of blocked lymph glands. In women, it also ensures a balanced hormone level.

Aroma therapy

Ylang-Ylang: This delicate oil, obtained from the blossoms of the ylang-ylang tree, is one of the best known aphrodisiacs. It has a relaxing effect and, at the same time, makes you conscious of subtle sensual sensations. Its sweet fragrance makes you feel safe and encourages you to entrust yourself to the flow of your feelings. Dammed-up feelings or turbulent emotions are dissolved and carried away with this fragrance.

Sandalwood: In the Far East, sandalwood oil was often used to increase sexual energy and to elevate union with the beloved partner to the level of a spiritual experience. Moreover, it stimulates the imagination and awakens the joy of being creatively active. The vibrations of sandalwood oil integrate the spiritual energies on all levels of thinking, feeling and acting.

The form of Yoga that works
primarily through the second chakra

Tantra Yoga: Tantra sees nature as the play between the female and male energies of Shakti and Shiva, who bring forth the visible world in a never-ending dance of Creation.

In Tantra, union with this "cosmic sexuality" is strived for by opening our senses, refining and heightening sexual experience and helping us to accept life.

The Third Chakra

*Manipura Chakra,
also called the Solar Plexus Chakra
or the Navel Center.
The terms Spleen, Stomach and
Liver Chakra are also used*

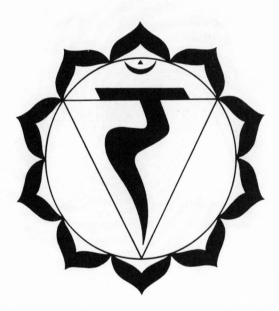

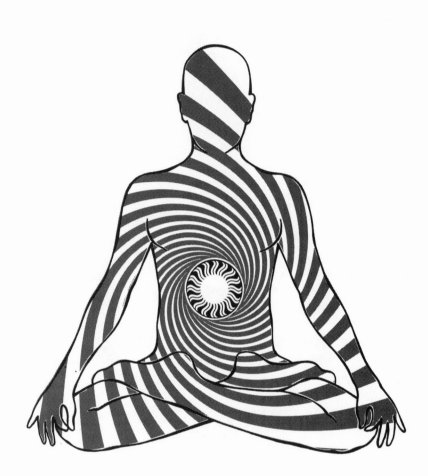

The third chakra is located approximately two fingerbreadths above the navel. It opens towards the front.

The Third Chakra and Its Associated Characteristics

Color: Yellow to golden

Associated element: Fire

Sense: Sight

Symbol: 10-petalled lotus

Basic principle: Shaping of being

Associated parts of the body: Lower back, abdomen, digestive system, stomach, liver, spleen, gallbladder, autonomic nervous system.

Associated gland: Pancreas (liver)
The pancreas plays an important part in the digestion of food. It secretes the hormone insulin, which regulates the amount of blood sugar in the system, as well as carbohydrate metabolism. The enzymes which are secreted by the pancreas are important for the balance of fats and proteins.

Associated astrological signs and planets:
Leo/Sun: Warmth, strength, abundance, striving for recognition, power and social status.
Sagittarius/Jupiter: Affirmation of life experience, growth and expansion, synthesis, wisdom, wholeness.
Virgo/Mercury: Classification, analysis, conformity. Selfless serving and devotion.
Mars: Energy and activity, willingness to act, self-assertion.

Purpose and function
of the third chakra

The third chakra is referred to by a number of terms. Accordingly, opinions diverge opinions about its location. In fact, we are dealing with a main chakra with several secondary chakras, but these are so closely related in their functions that they can be considered as one main chakra. Thus the functions of the third chakra are highly complex. It is assigned to the element of fire, and fire stands for light, warmth, energy and activity, and, on a spiritual plane, purification.

The solar plexus chakra represents our sun, our power center. Here we absorb the solar energy which nurtures our ethereal body, thereby vitalizing and maintaining our physical body. In the third chakra we enter into active contact with people and the material world. This is the part of our body from which our emotional energy radiates. Our relations with others, our likes and our dislikes and the ability to enter into a long-term relationship are for the most part controlled by this center.

For the ordinary person, the third chakra represents the foundation of his or her personality. Here we find our social identity and seek to confirm it, either by personal assertion, the will to achieve, a striving for power, or adaptation to social patterns.

The most important task of the third chakra consists of purifying the desires and wishes of the lower chakras, consciously controlling and using their creative energy and, finally, allowing the spiritual richness of the higher chakras to manifest in the material world as a means of achieving the greatest possible fulfillment on all levels of being.

It is directly connected to the astral body, which is also known as the center of our wishes and desires, and is the carrier of our emotions. Here the vital desires, wishes and feelings of the lower chakras are digested, so to speak, and transformed into a higher energy pattern that, in conjunction with the energies of the higher chakras, shapes our being.

The corresponding principle on the physical level is manifest in the liver. In combination with the digestive system, the liver fulfills the task of analyzing food once it has been ingested, separating the useful from the useless and transforming the former into usable substances before passed it on to the appropriate parts of our body.

The acceptance and integration of our feelings, wishes and experiences help the third chakra to relax and open up, thus increasing our inner light and illuminating our situation in life.

The general state of our moods depends to a large extent on how much light we permit to shine within ourselves. We feel enlightened, full of joy and inner richness when the third chakra is opened. If it is blocked or disturbed, we feel gloomy and somewhat unbalanced. Simultaneously, we project the same sensations into the world about us, so that life either seems bright or dark to us. It is the amount of light within us which determines the clearness of our vision and the quality of what we see.

Through increasing integration and inner wholeness, the third chakra gradually transforms the yellow light of intellectual understanding into the golden light of wisdom and abundance.

Through the solar plexus chakra we also directly perceive the vibrations of other people and react accordingly. If we are confronted with negative vibrations, a sudden contraction of the third chakra will warn us of potential danger. This is a temporary protective measure which becomes superfluous when our inner light is strong enough to envelope our body like a protective sheath.

Harmonious functioning

A harmoniously functioning and open third chakra creates a feeling of peace and inner harmony with your Self, life in general and your place in life in particular. You can accept yourself completely, and also respect the feelings and character traits of others.

You possess a natural capacity to accept your feelings, your wishes and what you experience in life, to see them "in the right light" and recognize them as a necessary part of your development. Thus you can integrate your feelings, wishes and experiences in such a way that they lead to wholeness.

All your actions are automatically in harmony with the cosmic laws of natural balance that apply to the entire universe and all human beings. When your actions contribute to the development of spiritual and material riches in both yourself and your neighbors, you are contributing to overall evolution. You are full of light and energy, and the light within you also envelops your body. It protects you from negative vibrations and radiates into your environment.

If your inner eye chakra and your crown chakra are also open, you recognize that all visible matter consists of varying light vibrations. Your wishes are fulfilled spontaneously because you are so closely connected to the energy of light in all things that you attract everything you are in search of.

You therefore live in the knowledge that abundance is your birthright and a divine heritage.

Disharmonious functioning

When your third chakra is one-sidedly active or malfunctioning, you want to manipulate everything in accordance with your own wishes, you want to control your inner and outer worlds, to conquer and exercise power. Nonetheless, you are driven by an inner restlessness and discontent. You probably experienced a lack of acceptance during your childhood years and adolescence. Therefore you were unable to develop a genuine sense of your own worth, and as a result seek the recognition and satisfaction you cannot find within yourself in the material world. You develop an enormous urge to be active in order to cover up your nagging feelings of inadequacy and shortcomings. You are in need of inner serenity and find it difficult to simply let go of things and relax.

Acceptance and material well-being are of primary importance for you, and perhaps you are quite successful in obtaining them.

Your attitude that nothing is impossible lets you suppress any manifestation of feeling as an undesirable or even bothersome phenomenon. As a consequence, your emotions are stopped-up. But occasionally they break through this wall of control and defense like a flood, making it impossible for you to channel them correctly. You get highly upset easily, but your agitation is an expression of all the anger you have swallowed over a long period of time.

One day you will finally have to acknowledge that striving for material wealth and recognition cannot provide you with true long-term satisfaction.

Insufficient functioning

Inadequate functioning of the third chakra often makes you feel dejected and discouraged. You see obstacles everywhere, obstacles that prevent the fulfillment of your desires.

The free unfolding of your personality was probably strongly curtailed when you were a child. Since you were afraid to lose the approval of your parents and teachers, you held back the expression of your emotions almost entirely and suppressed much more than you were able to "digest". This caused "emotional ashes" to pile up, which are now smothering the fiery energy of the solar plexus chakra and robbing your thoughts and actions of spontaneity and strength.

Even today you are trying to win acceptance and approval by conforming, but all you achieve is rejection and insufficient integration of your own vital desires and emotions. When faced with a difficult situation, you feel queasy and uncertain, or you get so nervous that your actions become haphazard and disorganized.

If possible, you would prefer to shut yourself off from all new challenges in life. Unusual experiences scare you, and you really do not feel capable of coping with the so-called "struggle for survival".

Possibilities for cleansing and activating the third chakra

Experiencing nature

Golden sunlight corresponds to the light, warmth and energy of the solar plexus chakra. If you consciously open yourself to its influence, it will revitalize these same qualities within you.

The contemplation of a ripe field of wheat bathed in the light of the sun conveys an experience of manifest abundance, a counterpart of the sun's warmth and radiant power.

If you look at a sunflower, you will see spiralling patterns in the unity of its intricate rosette, while the petals stream out golden light from this heart. By immersing yourself in the contemplation of this natural mandala, you will learn that within the inner experience of oneness exists a well-ordered and dance-like movement that radiates outward with energy and joy, yet gently and in a graceful way.

Sound therapy

Music: The third chakra is activated by fiery rhythms. Orchestral music with its harmonious interaction of sounds is suitable for harmonizing the energy of the solar plexus chakra. In the case of hyperactivity in this center, any type of relaxing music which leads you to your inner center will help calm you down.

Vowel: An open "o" as in the word "God" is related to the solar plexus chakra, and should be sung in E. The "o" sound produces a circular movement which is directed towards the outside. It stimulates the manifestation of being from within an inner wholeness. The open "o" also inclines itself towards the "a" of the heart chakra, thus entailing expanse, abundance and joy.

Mantra: RAM

Color therapy

A clear and sunny yellow activates and reinforces the functioning of the third chakra. The yellow color strengthens our nerves and thoughts, but it also stimulates contact and interaction with others. It compensates feelings of inner fatigue, creates joy and cheerful relaxation. Should you be too passive or dreamy, a clear yellow will help you to become actively involved with life. Moreover it aids digestion, both on a physical and spiritual plane.

A golden hue will clarifies and relax in cases of psychological problems or illness. It strengthens mental activity and stimulates the kind of wisdom that grows out of experience.

Gemstone therapy

Tiger's-eye: The tiger's-eye supports inner and outer vision. It sharpens our mind and helps us to recognize our own faults and act accordingly.

Amber: Amber provides us warmth and confidence. Its solar energy guides us on our way to greater joy and clearer light. It conveys new insights and teaches us how to realize our own Self in life. Thus, amber also brings us success in our undertakings.
On the physical level it cleanses and purifies the organism, helps balance the digestive system and the endocrine glands, and lastly cleans and fortifies the liver.

Topaz: The gold colored topaz fills us with the radiant energy and the warming light of the sun. It enriches us with greater consciousness, alertness, clearness, joy and vividness. Moreover, it carries away emotional burdens and gloomy thoughts. This may help you overcome anxiety and depression. Moreover, the topaz strengthens and stimulates the entire body and aids mental and physical digestion.

Citrine: The citrine produces a general feeling of well-being, warmth, vividness, security and trust. It helps you digest what you experience and transform intuitive perceptions into conscious action. It also attracts inner and outer abundance and helps you achieve your goals.

On the physical plane it helps excrete toxic substances and cure digestion problems and diabetes. Additionally, it revitalizes the blood and the nerves.

Aroma therapy

Lavender: Lavender oil has a calming, relaxing effect on hyperactive third chakras. Its gentle, warm vibrations help "digest" and dissolve dammed up emotions.

Rosemary: The tangy oil extracted from the rosemary plant is particularly appropriate in the case of an insufficiently functioning solar plexus chakra. Its stimulating and refreshing influence helps overcome inertia and fosters readiness for action.

Bergamot: The vibrations of the oil extracted from the fruits of the bergamot tree carry a great deal of light within them. Its fresh and lemon-like fragrance strengthens our life energies and gives us self-confidence and self-assurance.

The form of Yoga that works primarily through the third chakra

Karma Yoga: Karma Yoga helps us achieve selflessness in our actions, to no longer think of their possible results and our personal gains. Through Karma Yoga we open ourselves to the Divine Will and bring our actions into harmony with the natural cosmic energy of Creation.

The Fourth Chakra

Anahata Chakra,
also known as the Heart Chakra
or the Heart Center

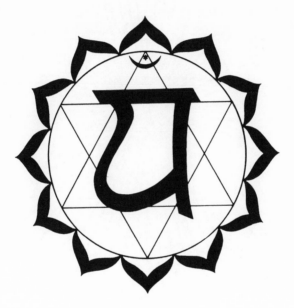

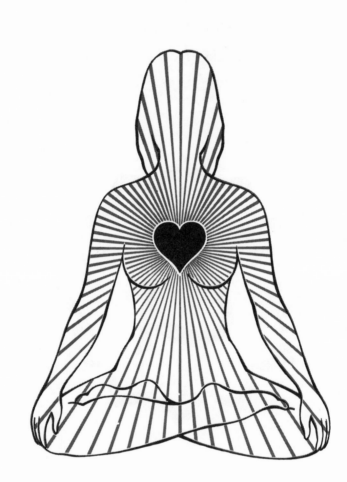

The fourth chakra is located in the center of the breast at the height of the heart.
It opens towards the front.

The Fourth Chakra and its Associated Characteristics

Color: Green, but also pink and gold

Associated element: Air

Sense: Touch

Symbol: 12-petalled lotus

Basic principle: Devotion, self-abandon

Associated parts of the body: Heart, upper back, including the thorax and the thoracic cavity, the lower area of the lungs, the blood and the blood circulation system, the skin.

Associated gland: Thymus.
The thymus gland regulates growth and controls the lymphatic system. It also has the function of stimulating and strengthening the immune system.

Associated astrological planets and signs:
Leo/Sun: Emotional warmth, sincerity, generosity.
Libra/Venus: Contact, love, striving for harmony. Augmentation of the Self.
Saturn: Overcoming the individual ego, thus making selfless love possible.

Purpose and function of the fourth chakra

The heart chakra is the center of the entire chakra system. It connects the three lower physical and emotional centers to the three higher mental and spiritual centers. The hexagon as its symbol clearly illustrates how the energies of the three lower and the three higher chakras mutually permeate each other. The fourth chakra is assigned to the element air and to the sense of touch. This indicates flexibility of the heart, the ability to establish contact and the willingness to be touched and at the same time be in touch with all things. Here we find the capability to empathize with others and sympathize with them, and to attune ourselves and join in with the cosmic vibrations. Through the same energy center we perceive beauty in nature as well as the harmony to be found in music, the visual arts and poetry. In the fourth chakra images, words and sounds are transformed into feelings.

The purpose of the heart chakra is to achieve perfect union through love. All yearning for deep, intimate contact, for oneness, harmony and love, even when these feelings come to us in the guise of sorrow, pain, fear of separation or loss of love, etc., is expressed via the heart chakra. In its pure and completely opened state, the fourth chakra forms the center of the true, unconditional love which exists only for its own sake and which therefore can neither be possessed nor lost. When connected with the higher chakras, this love transforms itself into Bhakti, the Divine Love which makes us aware of the Divine presence in all Creation and guides us to unity with this heart of all things in the universe. On its way toward achieving this goal, our heart must learn to love, understand and accept our own personality, the prerequisite to saying "yes" to others and life in general.

Once we have accepted that all our experiences, wishes and emotions have a deeper sense, and that their purpose is to lead us back through different steps of learning to an all-embracing order, we find in the fourth chakra a loving acceptance that all feelings and expressions of life come from the longing for love and union with life, and that in the final analysis, they, too, are an expression of love.

With every negation and rejection we regenerate separation and negativity, whereas positive and loving acceptance, a conscious "yes", produce vibrations in which negative forms of expression or feelings cannot survive. Perhaps you have already noticed that intense feelings of grief, anger or despair can be neutralized when you give them your loving, unbiased and undivided attention. If not, just try it occasionally.

If you suffer from pain or illness, giving the afflicted organ or part of the body your loving attention can accelerate recuperation enormously. With our heart chakra we therefore possess a great potential for transformation and healing, for others as well as ourselves. If we learn to love and fully accept all parts of our personality from the depths of our heart, we can be transformed or healed completely. This same love is the prerequisite for a fulfilling love for others, for compassion, understanding and an expansive joy that includes all life.

The energy of the heart chakra streams out extremely strongly, and an open heart chakra can have a spontaneous healing or transforming influence on others. However, in cases of conscious, deliberate healing, the inner eye chakra has to be part of the process.

The heart chakra radiates in the colors green, pink and sometimes gold. Green is the color of healing, sympathy and harmony. If an enlightened person (someone who is capable of "seeing" the aura) perceives a clear light green in a person's heart chakra, this indicates a well-developed capability to heal, while a golden aura, interwoven with pink, shows a person who lives in pure and selfless love of the Divine.

The heart chakra is often referred to as the seat of our deepest and most vivid feelings of love. Through this energy center we can also establish contact with the universal part of our soul, that spark of the Divine within us. The heart chakra also plays a decisive role in refining the perception that accompanies the opening of the Third Eye or brow chakra, for it is the devotion of the heart that makes us receptive to the subtler aspects of Creation. Thus the higher capabilities of the brow chakra develop concurrently with the unfolding of the heart chakra.

For this reason, many spiritual disciplines or schools in East and West concentrate particularly on the opening of the heart chakra.

Harmonious functioning

A completely open heart chakra that works together with all the other chakras in harmony will transform you into a channel for Divine love. The energies of your heart can change the world about you, and unite, reconcile or even heal the people in your surroundings. You radiate natural warmth, sincerity and happiness. This opens the hearts of the people around you, inspires confidence and creates joy. Compassion and the willingness to help come perfectly naturally to you.

Your feelings are free of inner disturbances, conflicts, doubts or uncertainty. You love for love's sake, motivated by the joy of giving, and do not expect to gain anything in the process. You feel safe and comfortable with all Creation. You put your heart into everything you do.

The love in your heart also makes you aware of the cosmic game of separation and renewed union taking place in all manifest life, maintained in this and permeated by Divine Love and harmony. Your own experience has taught you that longing for reunification with the Divine is rooted in separation from the Divine aspect of life and the sorrow resulting from this separation. To experience the infinite joy which grows out of true love of God, separation must take place first.

Through this "wisdom of the heart" you view worldly and personal happenings in a new light. The love in your heart spontaneously supports all efforts that help love for God and his Creation grow and prosper. You recognize that all beings, both sentient and non-sentient, live in your heart. No longer will you look at life from a distance and think that it has nothing to do with you. You see it as part of your own life.

The feeling of being alive grows so strongly within you that you begin to understand what "life" in its purest and most original form really signifies - an everlasting expression of Divine love and bliss.

Disharmonious functioning

A malfunctioning heart chakra may express itself in various ways. You might, for example, always want to be there for others and give freely, but without really being connected with the source of love. In secret - perhaps without being conscious of it or admitting to it - you always expect recognition and reassurance in return for all the "love" you give, and feel deeply disappointed when your efforts are not sufficiently appreciated.

It may also be that you feel strong and powerful enough to give away some of your strength. You are incapable, though, of accepting the love that others want to give you, and are unable to open yourself to receiving. Tenderness and softness make you feel embarrassed. Perhaps you tell yourself that you do not need the love others could give you. On the physical plane, this attitude is often accompanied by a widened, overly expanded thorax, which indicates an inner armor and a defense against all sorts of attack and pain.

Insufficient functioning

Inadequate functioning of the heart chakra makes you very vulnerable to injury and dependent on the love and affection of others. When you experience rejection, you are deeply hurt, especially since you had the courage to open yourself up. When this happens, you feel like withdrawing into your inner shell, are sad and depressed. You would like to give your love, but your fear of being rejected makes it impossible to find the right way of doing it. And from your point of view, this confirms your shortcomings and inability time and time again.

Perhaps you try to compensate for your lack of love by adopting extremely friendly and helpful ways. In doing so, you treat all people equally in a rather impersonal manner, without becoming genuinely involved. Whenever your heart is called for, you try to evade the situation, or shut yourself off because you are afraid of possible injury.

If your heart chakra is completely shut, this will express itself in coldness, indifference or even "heartlessness". In order to feel anything at all you require strong external stimulation. You are out of balance and suffer from depression.

Possibilities for cleansing and activating the fourth chakra

Experiencing nature

Every quiet walk through the unspoiled green countryside harmonizes your entire being through the heart chakra. Every single blossom conveys a message of love and innocent joy and lets the same qualities bloom in your heart. Pink-colored flowers are especially suitable for the gentle revitalization and healing of the heart chakra's energies.

A pink-colored sky with gossamer clouds brightens up and expands our hearts. Let the beauty and softness of the colors of this painting in the sky envelop you and carry you away.

Sound therapy

Music: Any type of classical, New Age or sacral music of the Eastern or Western tradition which has an edifying effect and makes your heart join in the dance of life is suitable for the heart chakra. It will awaken the power of love and influence it in a revitalizing and harmonizing way. Sacral or meditative dances which express the harmony and joy of Creation in their movements are also highly suitable.

Vowel: The vowel sound "ah" is assigned to the heart chakra and should be sung in F. The "ah" sound symbolizes direct awareness of our heart, as expressed in the exclamation "Ah!". It is the most open of all sounds and represents the greatest possible richness of expression available to the human voice. The "ah" sound expresses unbiased acceptance of all manifestation, the acceptance which brings forth love. It is the sound that babies, whose intellect is as yet unable to distinguish between "good" and "bad", use most frequently to "comment" on their experiences.

Mantra: YAM.

Color therapy

Green: The color of the meadows and forests of our planet provides us with harmony and compassion and makes us receptive to reconciliation. We feel empathy and experience inner peace and serenity. Additionally, green has a regenerating effect on the body, mind and soul, and provides us with new energy.

Pink: The gentle, tender vibrations of the color pink can loosen tension in our heart, awaken feelings of love and tenderness and bring back a childlike feeling of happiness. These vibrations also stimulate creative activity.

Gemstone therapy

Rose Quartz: The soft, pink-colored light of the rose quartz encourages gentleness, tenderness and love. It envelops your soul in loving vibrations that heal the wounds of your heart caused by hardness, lack of consideration or carelessness, and opens your soul so that it is able to give and receive love more freely.

The rose quartz teaches you to accept and love yourself, and opens your heart for all expressions of love and tenderness within yourself, in others and in all Creation. It makes you receptive for the beauty of music, poetry, painting and other art forms and enlivens your imagination and creative power of expression.

Tourmaline: The pinkish-red tourmaline leads you out of narrow emotional structures and opens and expands your heart. It makes you conscious of the joy-bringing aspect of love and connects you with the female manifestation of Divine Love as expressed in the beauty of Creation, in innocent joy, spiritual dance or play. Thus it integrates the various expressions of Divine and worldly love.

Pink tourmalines edged in green, which are often available as cut slices, are of particular value, since they unite the expansive qualities of the pinkish-red tourmaline with the healing, harmonizing vibration of the color green.

Kunzite: The kunzite combines the tender pink of higher love with the violet of the crown chakra which supports union with the Divine.

Kunzite opens your heart chakra to Divine Love and helps you develop your heart to the point of selflessness and perfection. It will make you straightforward and will always lead you back onto this path if ever you leave it.

Emerald: The emerald is the gemstone of all-embracing love, for it strengthens and deepens love on all levels. While providing you with peace and inner harmony, it will also tune you into the energies of nature. Furthermore, it challenges you to equal its brilliant light and shows you areas where this is not yet the case.

The emerald draws healing energies from the cosmos to the earth. It regenerates, rejuvenates, refreshes and relaxes.

Jade: The soft, green light of jade brings peace, harmony, wisdom of the heart, fairness and modesty. Jade relaxes our heart and makes us calm, lets us discover and experience the beauty of all nature and thus enhances our appreciation of and love for all Creation. Jade will bring relief if you are fidgety and restless, and will help you sleep peacefully and have pleasant dreams.

Aroma therapy

Attar of roses: No other fragrance has such a harmonizing effect on our well-being as the precious attar of roses. Its gentle, loving vibrations soothe and heal the wounds of our heart. They awaken our perception of love, beauty and harmony everywhere in Creation. A deep joy and a readiness for dedication enter our heart. Attar or oil of roses also induces stimulation and refinement of sensual pleasures, and at the same time helps transform them into transcendental love.

The form of yoga that works primarily through the fourth chakra

Bhakti Yoga: Bhakti Yoga is the way which leads to the realization of the Divine through devotion and love of God. Devotees deepen and intensify their feelings and direct them towards God. They relate everything to Him, perceive Him in all things and are transfigured in their love for Him.

The Fifth Chakra

Vishuddha Chakra,
also referred to
as the Neck or Throat Chakra,
or as the Communication Center

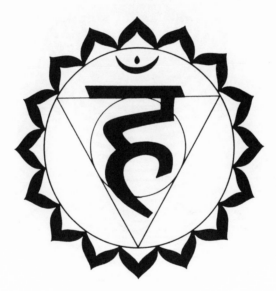

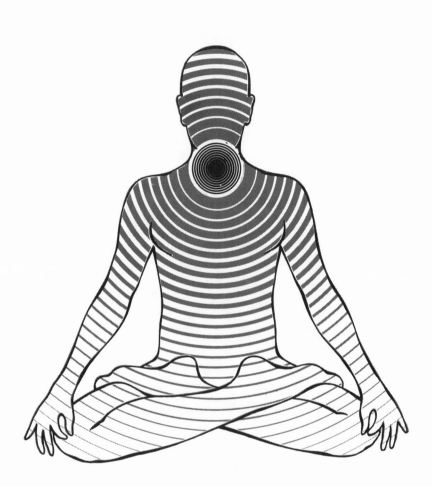

The fifth chakra is located between the depression in the neck and the larynx.
It starts at the cervical vertebra and opens towards the front.

The Fifth Chakra
and its Associated Characteristics

Color: Pale blue, also silver or greenish blue.

Associated element: Ether.

Sense: Hearing.

Symbols: 16-petalled lotus.

Basic principle: Resonance of being.

Associated parts of the body: Neck, throat and jaw. Ears, voice, trachea, bronchial tubes, upper lungs, esophagus, arms.

Associated gland: Thyroid.
The thyroid gland plays an important part in the growth of the skeleton and inner organs. It governs the balance between physical and spiritual growth and via our metabolism regulates the manner and the speed of the transformation of food into energy, as well as the use of this energy. Moreover, it controls the iodine metabolism and the balance of calcium in blood and tissues.

Associated astrological planets and signs:
Gemini/Mercury: Communication, interchange of knowledge and experience.
Mars: Active self-expression.
Taurus/Venus: Feeling for form and space.
Aquarius/Uranus: Divine inspiration, conveying of knowledge and higher wisdom, independence.

Purpose and function
of the fifth chakra

The throat chakra is the center of the human capacity of expression, communication and inspiration. It is connected to a smaller secondary chakra which has its seat in the neck and opens to the back. These two energy centers are often viewed as one. In its function the neck chakra is so closely related to the throat chakra that we have integrated it into the interpretation of the fifth chakra.

The fifth chakra also constitutes an important link between the lower chakras and the crown center. It serves as a bridge between our thoughts and feelings, our impulses and reactions. At the same time, it communicates the contents of all chakras to the external world. Through the throat chakra we express everything alive within us - our laughing and crying, our feelings of love and happiness, anxiety and aggressiveness, our intentions and desires as well as our ideas, knowledge and perceptions of inner worlds.

The element assigned to the throat chakra is ether. In Yoga teachings it is regarded as the basic element which forms the lower chakras: earth, water, fire and air. Ether is also the medium of sound, of the spoken word in general, as well as the divine word of Creation. It is, to put it briefly, the communicating element or the mediator of information on all levels of being.

Communication of our inner life primarily takes place through the spoken word, and also through gestures and creative forms of expression, such as music, the visual and performing arts, dancing, etc. In the throat chakra the creativity of the sacral chakra joins with the energies of the other chakras, and the ether shapes these energies into the form in which it is communicated to the external world.

However, we only can express that which we find in ourselves, and thus one of the tasks of the fifth chakra is to provide us a certain inner distance and thus enable us to reflect on our thoughts and actions. The more we develop the throat chakra, the more we become conscious of our mental body and the more we are able to distinguish between the functions of the latter and those of the emotional, ethereal and physical bodies. As a result, our thoughts are no longer dominated by feelings and physical sensations, which makes objective cognition possible.

Ether is also defined as Akasha, the astral light where all the events, actions, thoughts and feelings that have occurred since the beginning of time are recorded. If we become expansive and open like boundless space and the infinite sky, we will be granted the deepest level of knowledge and insight. The light blue color of ether is also that of the throat chakra. The best way of achieving such deep knowledge is to become calm and listen to our inner and outer space. The sensual function of hearing is assigned to the fifth chakra. Here we open our ears and listen to the manifest and concealed voices of Creation. And it is here that we perceive our own inner voice, and enter into contact with our inner spirit and receive its inspiration. We also develop an unshakable confidence in our personal higher guidance. We become conscious of our own real mission in life, our Dharma. We recognize that our inner worlds and subtle planes of being are as real as the material world; we are capable of absorbing and transmitting information from the subtler spheres and higher dimensions of reality. This divine inspiration becomes a basic element of our self-expression.

Through the fifth chakra we find our own, individual expression of perfection on all levels of being.

Harmonious functioning

With a completely open throat chakra you express your feelings, thoughts and inner knowledge freely and without fear, and are also capable of revealing your weaknesses or showing your strengths. Your inner honesty towards yourself and others is expressed by your upright posture.

You possess the ability to fully express yourself with your entire personality. If appropriate, you can also remain silent and listen to others with all your heart and understanding. Your speech is imaginative and colorful, yet at the same time perfectly clear. It communicates your intentions in the most effective way for achieving the fulfillment of your wishes. Your voice is full and melodious. When faced with difficulties and resistance, you remain true to yourself and are able to say "no", if that's what you mean. Other people's opinions do not sway or manipulate you; instead, you maintain your independence, freedom and self-determination. Being free of prejudices and possessing great inner spaciousness, you are open to the reality of subtle dimensions. From them you receive the guidance of your inner voice, which leads you on your way through life. You trustingly place yourself in the hands of this guidance. You recognize that all manifestations in Creation have their own individual message. They tell you about their lives, their parts in the universal game, and about their striving for wholeness and light. You possess the capability of communicating directly with life from other spheres of being, and whenever it appears appropriate, you pass the knowledge you have gained on to others, without fearing their reactions and opinions. All the means you employ for creative expression can convey wisdom and truth.

Out of your inner independence and the free expression of your entire being arises deep joy and a feeling of completeness and integrity.

Disharmonious functioning

If the energies in your throat chakra are blocked, this will interfere with the communication between mind and body. This can occur in two different ways. Either you find it difficult to reflect about your feelings and therefore often express your unresolved emotions in thoughtless actions. Or else you may shut yourself off inside your intellect, and deny your emotions a right to live. The only feelings you permit are those which have passed through the filter of your self-judgement and which do not contradict the judgement of the people around you. An unconscious feeling of guilt and your own inherent fears prevent you from seeing and showing your true Self, from expressing your deepest thoughts, feelings and needs freely. Instead, you try to cover them up with a multitude of words and gestures which conceal your true Being.

Your language is either blatant and coarse or cool and businesslike. You may stutter. Your voice is comparatively loud and your words lack deeper meaning. You do not permit yourself any appearance of weakness, but instead constantly try to appear strong at all costs. As a result, you probably place yourself under great pressure. It might be that life's demands weigh too heavily upon your shoulders. In this case you assume a defensive mode, raise your shoulders and pull in your neck to protect yourself against additional burdens and arm yourself against a new attack.

Disharmonious functioning of the fifth chakra can also be found in people who abuse their expressive capability in order to manipulate others, or to draw attention to themselves with an uninterrupted flow of words.

As a rule, people with blocked energies in the throat chakra do not have access to the subtle dimensions of being, as they lack the openness, the inner expanse and the independence which are prerequisites for perceiving these spheres.

Nevertheless, there is the possibility that you possess deep, inner knowledge. You are simply afraid to live or express it because you fear the judgement of others, and isolation. This deep knowledge may force its way into the open in the form of poems, paintings or other means of spontaneous expression, but you share them with others very reluctantly. Your spiritual energies may get bogged down in your head. Then their transforming powers will have difficulty finding their way to your emotions, and the energies of the lower chakras will not provide the upper chakras with the power and stability they need to realize inner spirituality in your life.

Insufficient functioning

Insufficient functioning of your throat chakra hinders your capability to show and express yourself. You hold back your inner Self completely; you are shy, quiet and withdrawn, and when you talk it is only about trivialities regarding your external life.

If you do try to express your deeper thoughts and feelings, you quickly get a lump in your throat and your voice sounds forced. Here the symptom of stuttering is even more frequent than in cases of disharmonious functioning. With regard to others you feel uncertain and afraid of their judgement, and you frequently don't really know what you want. You are out of touch with the messages of your soul and do not trust your intuitive powers.

If you do not develop your fifth chakra, a certain stiffness will set in. The space behind your self-built walls, the space where you spend most of your time, where you express your potential, is small and restrictive because you only accept the external world as valid reality.

Possibilities for cleansing and activating the fifth chakra

Experiencing nature

The light, transparent blue of a cloudless sky stimulates a reaction within your throat chakra. In order to completely absorb the azure hue, lie down on the ground and relax, opening your inner being to the boundless expanse of the firmament. You will feel how your mind opens and clears, and how the contractions and rigidities in your throat chakra and its sphere of influence gradually dissolve. Now your heart is ready to receive the "messages" of the Divine.

The reflection of the blue sky in a clear stretch of water will have a widening and liberating effect on your feelings, and the soft sound of the waves will make you aware of your hidden emotions and what they have to tell you. If you let yourself be completely permeated by the vibrating energies of sky and water, your mind and feelings will augment each other perfectly.

Sound therapy

Music: Any kind of music or song rich in high tones as well as meditative dancing or singing have a particularly stimulating influence. In order to harmonize and relax the throat chakra, listen to peaceful New Age music with echo effects. It liberates, widens and opens the "inner ear".

Vowel: The vowel sound "eh", which should be sung in G, revives the fifth chakra. If you sing from "ah" to "e" very, very slowly, you will notice that an "eh" emerges at a certain brief point. Just as the throat connects the head to the body, so too the "eh" of the throat chakra combines and connects the heart ("a") and the mind ("e"), channelling their energies to the outside. When you sing "eh", you will notice that it requires the most pressure of all the chakra sounds, thus underlining the ex"pression" of your fifth chakra.

Mantra: HAM.

Color therapy

A light and clear shade of blue is assigned to the throat chakra. This color creates calmness and expanse and opens you up to spiritual inspiration.

Gemstone therapy

Aquamarine: The light blue color of the aquamarine resembles the sea reflecting a cloudless sky. It therefore helps convert your soul into a mirror reflecting the infinite expanse of your spirit. It also stimulates communication with your innermost being and brings light and clearness into the hidden reaches of your soul. Its vibrations fill your soul with purity, freedom and spaciousness, making it receptive to visionary clearness and intuitive understanding. The aquamarine also helps you to express this knowledge freely and creatively. Under its influence your soul can become a channel of selfless love and healing power.

Turquoise: Within the color of the turquoise we find a reunion between the blue of the sky and the green of the earth. Thus the turquoise combines the high ideals of the spirit with the primordial life energy of our planet. It helps express spiritual ideas and knowledge and integrate them into life on earth. Moreover, it absorbs positive energy and protects the body and our soul against negative influences.

Chalcedony: The white-blue chalcedony has positive effects on the thyroid gland. It exerts a calming and balancing influence on the mind and reduces irritability and hypersensitivity. Through its relaxing influence it opens the door to inner inspiration and stimulates creative self-expression through speech or writing.

Aroma therapy

Sage: The tangy fragrance of sage sends healing vibrations into the "seat of language". It loosens tensions in the throat chakra and lets us express what we have to say in a harmonious and energetic way, helping us to effectively communicate the inner messages of the soul.

Eucalyptus: The refreshing fragrance of eucalyptus oil clears and widens the fifth chakra. Its vibrations open us to our inner voice, and lends creativity and naturalness to our means of communication.

The form of Yoga that works primarily through the fifth chakra

Mantra Yoga: Mantras are meditative incantations that reflect certain aspects of the Divine. They are either silently recited, sung out loud or chanted. By repeating a mantra, thoughts and feelings are gradually transformed, thus attuning the devotee to the Divine cosmic power expressed by the given mantra.

Transcendental Meditation forms an exception in this respect. It consists of a technique which enables the devotee to experience the mantra on increasingly fine and subtle levels of consciousness until he transcends even the most subtle aspects of the mantra, enabling him to experience the purest form of being. This process takes place several times during a session of Transcendental Meditation.

The Sixth Chakra

*Ajna Chakra,
also known as the Brow Chakra,
the Third Eye, the Eye of Wisdom,
the Inner Eye Chakra
or the Command Chakra*

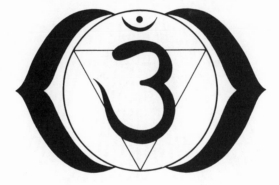

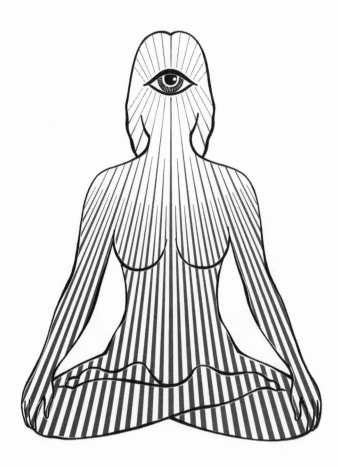

The sixth chakra is located a fingerbreadth above the bridge of the nose in the center of the forehead. It opens to the front.

The Sixth Chakra
and Its Associated Characteristics

Color: Indigo, also yellow or violet.

Sense: All senses, including extrasensory perception.

Symbols: 96-petalled lotus (2 x 48 petals)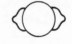

Basic principle: Knowledge of being

Associated parts of the body: Face, eyes, ears, nose, sinuses, cerebellum, central nervous system.

Associated gland: Pituitary (hypophysis).
The pituitary is sometimes referred to as the "master gland" because its secretional activities control the functions of the other glands. Like the conductor of an orchestra, it establishes the harmonious interaction of the other glands.

Associated astrological signs and planets:
Mercury: Intellectual cognition, rational thought.
Sagittarius/Jupiter: Holistic thought, realization of inner correlations.
Aquarius/Uranus: Divinely inspired thought, higher knowledge, flashes of intuition.
Pisces/Neptune: Imagination, intuition, access to inner truths through devotion.

Purpose and function of the sixth chakra

Conscious perception of Being takes place through the sixth chakra. It is the seat of our higher mental powers, our intellectual capacity to distinguish, our memory and our will. On the physical plane it is the highest center of command for the central nervous system.

Its actual color is a clear indigo blue, but yellow and violet shades are also to be found. These colors indicate different functions at various level of consciousness. Rational or intellectual thought may produce yellow radiation, while a clear dark blue color indicates intuition and holistic cognition. Extrasensory perception is shown in shades of violet.

Every realization in our lives is preceded by thoughts and projected images which in turn can be nurtured either by subconscious emotional patterns or a knowledge of reality. By mental power we are connected with the process of manifestation via the third eye. All knowledge manifest in Creation already exists, is contained in pure Being in the same way that a seed contains all the information the finished plant requires. Quantum physics refers to this sphere as the "standardized field" or the "area of the lowest stimulation of matter".

The creative process starts when Being resting in itself becomes conscious of its existence. An initial relationship between subject and object takes place, thus giving rise to duality. Being in its shapelessness manifests a first pattern of vibration.

On the basis of this first, primordial vibration each step forward in the development of awareness creates a new and differentiated pattern of vibration. Thus all levels of creation are contained in human life, from pure ethereal being to the densest of matter, and in turn are represented in the chakras with their various levels of vibrations. Thus the process of manifestation also takes place within and through us.

As the third eye is the seat of attainment of consciousness, it is here that we can manifest matter and dematerialize it. We are able to create new realities at the physical level and dissolve old ones.

As a rule, however, this process takes place automatically and without conscious action on our part. Most of the decisive thoughts in our lives are controlled by unresolved emotional patterns and programmed by our opinions and prejudices and by those of others. Our mind, therefore, is often not the master but the servant of the emotionally loaded thoughts that sometimes dominate us.

These thoughts also manifest into our lives, for what we perceive and experience outside is but a manifestation of our subjective reality.

By developing our consciousness and increasingly opening the third eye, we can control this process more consciously, and our imagination can create the energy for the fulfillment our wishes. In conjunction with an open heart chakra, we can send out healing energies, both close at hand and over long distances.

At the same time we can gain access to all levels of creation beyond physical reality. Knowledge of this reaches us in the form of intuition, clairvoyance or hypersensitive hearing or feeling. Things that we had only vaguely suspected before are now perceived clearly.

Harmonious functioning

Nowadays there are very few people with the completely opened third eye that always accompanies an advanced state of consciousness. However, in spite of incomplete development, the sixth chakra can function far more harmoniously than any of the other chakras. This expresses itself in an active mind and advanced intellectual skills. The holistic pursuit of scientific research or the recognition of far-reaching philosophical truths may be a sign of a partly opened and harmoniously functioning third eye chakra.

You probably possess a well-developed capacity for visualization and the ability to comprehend many things intuitively. Your mind is composed, and at the same time open to mystic truths. You realize more and more that the world of appearances is but an allegory, a symbol of a spiritual principle manifested on the physical level. Idealism and phantasy are the key elements of your thinking. You possibly notice from time to time that your thoughts or ideas come true.

The more your third eye chakra develops, the more your thoughts are based on a direct inner awareness of reality. Increasing numbers of people are beginning to develop sixth chakra skills, such as clairvoyance or sharpened sensitivity at particular levels of being; others achieve temporary insight into other dimensions of reality, for instance during sleep or meditation.

It is, however, impossible for us to describe the entire range of skills and perceptions that an open third eye is capable of. Such an endeavor would fill many volumes and we would have to rely on the information of others. Nevertheless, we would like to give you a general idea of what lies ahead if you manage to develop your sixth chakra completely.

First of all, you will perceive the world in a new way. The limitations of rational thought will be totally transcended. Your thinking will be holographic and you will spontaneously integrate the information reaching you from different spheres of creation into your growing capability of all-awareness.

The material world will become transparent to you. Much as your consciousness serves as a mirror for the Divine, the material world will mirror the dance of energy that takes place on all subtle levels of being. Your extrasensory perception is so clear that you directly perceive the energies at work beneath the surface of external things. Furthermore, you can consciously control these energies and create your own forms of manifestation for them. Nonetheless, you will be constrained to set rules whose limits you cannot exceed, meaning that a natural order will always be maintained.

Your intuition and inner sight will open the way to all subtle planes of reality. You will recognize that there is an endless number of worlds between the planes of material creation and pure Being, and that they are inhabited by a large variety of life forms. A multifacetted drama of creation will take place before your inner eye, and there will seem to be no limit to ever-new forms and levels of reality. The sight of this divine "dance of creation" will fill you with profound awe.

Disharmonious functioning

The most frequent consequence of a disharmoniously functioning sixth chakra is "top-heaviness", i.e. overemphasis of the mental sphere. Your life is determined almost exclusively by reason and intellect. Since you are trying to organize all aspects of your life in an intellectual manner, you only accept what you perceive with your rational mind. Your intellectual skills may be quite well developed and you may possess the gift of keen analysis, but you are lacking a holistic way of seeing things and the capability of integrating all that you experience into a single cosmic law of natural balance.

You can easily become a victim of intellectual arrogance. The only things you accept are those that the mind can comprehend, that can be demonstrated and proven by scientific method. You reject spiritual insight as unscientific and unrealistic.

Another effect that a disharmoniously functioning third eye chakra can have is that you may attempt to influence human beings or events by the force of your mind, simply to demonstrate your power or to satisfy your personal needs. In this case, the solar plexus chakra is usually out of balance, and the heart and crown chakras are only developed to a slight degree. If your third eye is opened relatively wide in spite of its blockages, you might even succeed in this undertaking, although your intentions are contrary to the natural flow of life. But sooner or later you will be beset by a feeling of isolation and the satisfaction you strived for will not be long-lasting.

Another possible consequence of misdirected energies in the sixth chakra occurs when the base chakra (and thus the element that "grounds" you) is disturbed, and when the other chakras are not functioning harmoniously. Although you have access to the subtler levels of perception, it can happen that you do not grasp the true meaning of the images and information you receive. Due to unresolved emotional patterns, they get mixed up with your own imagination. These subjective images can become so strong and dominating that you begin to consider them to be the only truth. You project them onto the external world and thus in the final analysis lose touch with reality.

Insufficient functioning

If the flow of energies in the sixth chakra is blocked to a considerable degree, the only reality you will see and accept is that of the external, visible world. Your life is dominated by material desires, physical needs and unreflected emotions. You find spiritual reflection and discussion a strain and a waste of time, and you reject spiritual truths because you view them as products of senseless dreaming without any practical use. Your thoughts are orientated along the established lines of society.

You easily lose your head in demanding situations. You are probably also very forgetful. If your vision is impaired, an effect which often accompanies insufficient functioning of the sixth chakra, you should look within yourself more closely and get to know the areas that lie beneath the surface.

In extreme cases, your thinking will be muddled and confused, and completely determined by unresolved emotional patterns.

Possibilities for cleansing
and activating the sixth chakra

Experiencing nature

The third eye can be stimulated by the contemplation of the starry, deep blue night sky. This experience of nature opens your mind to the boundless expanses of all manifestation in all its immensely varied forms of expression. It gives you an idea of the subtle energies, structures and laws at work behind the visible plane of life, as are represented by the dance of the celestial bodies in the infinity of space .

Sound therapy

Music: You can utilize any sounds which relax and open your mind and which evoke images or feelings of cosmic dimensions. New Age music will be particularly suitable in this respect, but there are also pieces of Eastern and Western classical music (in the latter case particularly by Bach), which will also stimulate and harmonize the third eye chakra.

Vowel: This chakra is activated by the vowel-sound "e" (as in "easy"), which should be sung in A. It sets off an upward movement and represents the power of inspiration that leads to the new insights.

Mantra: KSHAM.

Color therapy

Transparent indigo has an opening and purifying effect on the sixth chakra. It provides the mind with inner calmness, clarity and depth, and strengthens and heals the senses as well as opening them to subtle levels of perception.

Gemstone therapy

Lapis lazuli: In the deep blue of the lapis lazuli we find golden inclusions of pyrite, scattered like stars in the sky at night. Lapis lazuli conveys a feeling of security within the cosmos to our soul. It leads the mind inwards, strengthens its energies and makes it recognize higher principles. By stimulating our intuition and inner sight it makes us realize the hidden meaning of the material world and the energies at work beyond it. It also fills us with deep joy at the miracles of life and the universe.

Indigo-blue sapphire: A clear, transparent sapphire opens our mind to cosmic knowledge and eternal truths and its vibrations have a purifying, transforming and renewing effect on our bodies and souls. It builds a bridge between the finite and the infinite and makes our consciousness flow with the stream of Divine Love and cognition. It also brings clarity to souls in search of truth on the spiritual path.

Sodalite: The dark blue sodalite purifies our mind and enables it to think more deeply. Its still radiance fills us with serenity and strengthens our nerves. It also helps dissolve obsolete patterns of thought and gives us the trust and energy necessary to stick to our opinions and apply our ideas and knowledge to everyday life.

Aroma therapy

Mint: The refreshing scent of mint dissolves blockages within the sphere of the third eye and helps rid oneself of old, confining thought patterns. It clears and brightens the mind and stimulates concentration.

Jasmin: Through the fine, flowery scent of jasmin our mind is opened to images and visions which carry the messages of deeper truth. Its vibrations sharpen our senses and combine the energies of the third eye chakra with those of the heart chakra.

Forms of Yoga
working primarily through the sixth chakra

Jnana Yoga: Jnana Yoga is the way of awareness based on the development of the mind's capacity to distinguish between the real and the unreal, the eternal and the transitory. The Jnana Yogi realizes that there is only one unalterable, everlasting and eternal reality: God. Through meditation and the power to differentiate, the devotee focuses exclusively on the Absolute until his or her mind becomes one with the unmanifested aspect of God.

Yantra Yoga: Yantras are pictorial symbols depicting geometrical forms which represent the divine Being in all its aspects. They serve as an aid to visualization. The person meditating becomes completely immersed in the depicted aspects and visualizes them within by inner contemplation.

The Seventh Chakra

Sahasrara Chakra
or Crown Chakra,
also known as the Vertex Center
or the 1,000-petalled Lotus

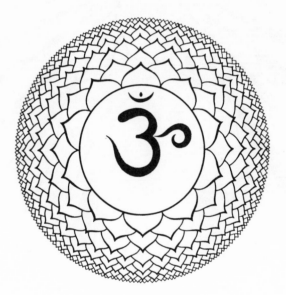

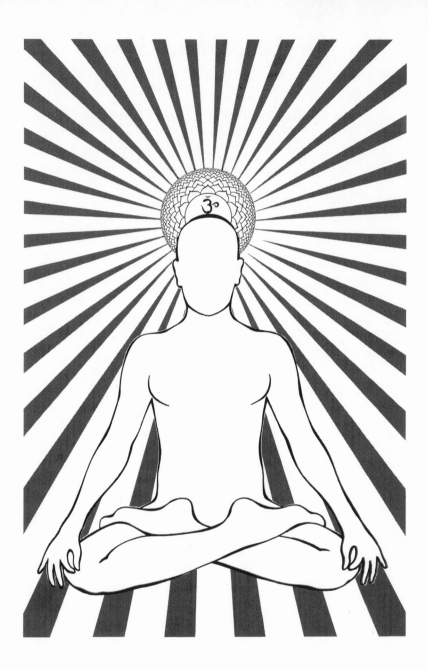

The seventh chakra is located at the middle of the head at its highest point.
It opens upward.

The Seventh Chakra
and Its Associated Characteristics

Color: Violet, also white and gold.

Symbol: 1,000-petalled lotus.

Basic principle: Purest Being.

Associated part of the body: Cerebrum.

Associated gland: Pineal body (epiphysis).
The influence of the epiphysis has not been conclusively determined by science. Most probably it effects our entire organism. A dysfunction of this gland results in premature sexual maturity.

Associated astrological signs and planets:
Capricorn/Saturn: Inner viewing, concentration on the essential, permeation of matter by Divine light.
Pisces/Neptune: Dissolution of limits, devotion, oneness with the Omnipresent Being.

Purpose and function
of the seventh chakra

The crown chakra is the seat of highest human perfection, and is often represented as hovering above the head. It glows in all colors of the rainbow, but the predominant color is violet. The outer blossom of this chakra consists of 960 petals. Inside we find a second blossom with 12 petals, glowing in white light interspersed with gold.

Just as all the colors of the spectrum are united in colorless light, the highest chakra unites in itself all the energies of the lower centers. It is the source and starting point for the manifestation of all other chakra energies. Here we are connected with the level of Being which contains all non-manifest forms and characteristics.

It is the place where we feel at home. From here we once started our journey into life, and to this place we will return at the end of our development. Here we live and experience unity with the primordial Divine principle of which we are all part. Our personal energy field becomes one with the universe.

Whatever we understood intellectually and later intuitively now reaches the point of complete comprehension. The awareness given to us by the seventh chakra goes far beyond the knowledge conveyed by the third eye chakra, for here we are no longer separated from the object of our perception. We experience the most varied expressions of Creation, i.e. our own bodies, as a play of divine consciousness of which we have become part.

The path to the unfolding of the seventh chakra is indicated in the color violet. Violet is the color of meditation and devotion. While we are able to consciously influence the activation of the six lower energy centers, in the case of the seventh all we can do is open ourselves and let things happen through us.

When the seventh chakra unfolds, any blockages remaining in the other six dissolve and their energies begin to vibrate at their highest possible frequencies. Each chakra works as a mirror of the Divine Being at its own particular level, and expresses the highest potential it is capable of.

As soon as the crown chakra is completely awakened, its task of absorbing cosmic energies comes to an end and it starts to radiate energy of its own accord. A lotus blossom reaches out, so to speak, to form a crown of pure light on the head.

Harmonious functioning

There are no blockages as such in the seventh chakra. It can only be developed to a greater or lesser extent.

When your crown chakra begins to open, you will experience more and more moments when the division between inner being and outer life recedes into the background. Your consciousness is completely calm and open, and you experience your real Self as being part of the omnipresent pure Being which contains all matter.

As the development of the crown chakra increases, these moments occur more frequently until they become permanent reality. When your Self is ready for this final step of enlightenment, it may happen quite suddenly. You will feel as if you have woken up from a long dream and that you are finally now beginning to live in reality. There will be no backward steps in your development. You have transformed yourself into an empty vessel, and the Divine Being fills this bowl to the rim. You realize you have found your true Self, the only permanent reality. Your individual ego has been transformed into a universal ego. You translate the purpose of the Creator into action in your behaviour, and the light you radiate opens the hearts of those receptive for the presence of the Divine. If you want to know something, you only have to direct your attention accordingly, because through your oneness with the divine Being everything exists within you. Creation is a game which takes place within your own boundless consciousness.

You realize that matter is nothing but a form of thought in the Divine Consciousness and does not really "exist" as such. All that you have accepted as real until now becomes an illusion. You experience the greatest emptiness - but this emptiness is identical with the greatest abundance, for it is life in its purest essence. And this divine essence is pure bliss.

During the years of the seven-year cycle in which you are particularly open to the energies of the crown chakra, you can develop a depth of insight and wholeness you would have considered previously impossible. Meditation and selfless devotion now provide you with insight into your Divine origin and help you experience a feeling of oneness. You should use this opportunity to dwell more within yourself.

In this context it is interesting to note that a baby's fontanel remains open for the first 9 to 24 months of its life. During this initial period of their lives on earth infants live in an awareness of undivided unity.

The characteristics of
a largely closed seventh chakra

As we have seen, the opening and harmonization of all the chakras described up to this point can provide us with a great deal of knowledge, experience and skills. Without the opening of the crown chakra, however, we will feel separated from abundance and wholeness, and will not be completely free of fear. It is this fear which always maintains some remnants of blockages within the chakras. Being unable to unfold their complete range of possibilities, the individual energies neither vibrate in complete harmony with the "dance of creation", nor in harmony with each other.

Unless you open yourself to spiritual truths during the years when the crown center can develop, you may experience feelings of uncertainty and a lack of purpose during this time. You should interpret these feelings as a hint to look inside yourself more frequently. You may also become conscious of a certain senselessness in your life, or the fear of death may visit you more often. Perhaps you will try to control these nagging feelings by escaping into excessive activity, or you m ay burden yourself with new responsibilities in order to make yourself indispensable. Quite often, people in this condition fall ill, which compels them to rest. If you ignore these messages, you may get stuck into a life of superficiality and limit the potential of your Self to develop.

Possibilities for cleansing
and activating the seventh chakra

Experiencing nature

Time spent alone on the peak of a very high mountain is the best way of helping your seventh chakra to open up, for here you are far away from your earthly cares and can easier let go of the events of your personal life. This and the closeness to the heavens helps you experience a feeling of space and boundlessness.

Sound therapy

Music: The best music for the crown chakra is silence. In states of complete silence our whole being becomes awake and receptive for the Divine sound that resounds through Creation, representing the power of love and the harmony of all manifestation. Any kind of music that will leads you into this silence or prepare you for it is also suitable.

Vowel: The sound "m", which is regarded as a vowel in India, opens the crown chakra. It resembles an endless humming vibration without limit or structure and should be sung in B. It represents unity and the pure, unformed and unlimited consciousness that contains all matter in its latent form.

Mantra: OM.

Color therapy

Violet and white have an opening and expanding effect on the crown chakra.

The violet color brings about a transformation of mind and soul and opens both to spiritual dimensions of being. It dissolves blockages and can guide us towards an experience of cosmic unity.

White contains all of the colors of the spectrum. It integrates the different levels of life to a higher unity and opens our souls to divine light, knowledge and healing.

Gemstone therapy

Amethyst: The red fire of activity and the blue light of receptiveness, silence and space unite into a greater potency in the amethyst. The stone transmits a vivid calmness which dissolves fear and disharmony while providing us with trust in and devotion to the energies of the universe. It guides our minds to the infinite, and stimulates meditation and inspiration.

Rock crystal: The rock crystal guides us on our path to the greater wholeness which contains and combines the colorful variety of life. It brings clearness and light to our minds and souls and stimulates spiritual cognition. It helps our souls to merge with the universal spirit, dissolves congestions and blockages, and provides us with new energy and protection.

Aroma therapy

Olibanum: It is no coincidence that the classical incense burnt in religious ceremonies consists of the resin of the olibanum tree. Its fragrance has a revitalizing effect on mind and soul and purifies the atmosphere. Everyday life fades into the background, religious convictions deepen and the souls becomes a willing vessel for the Divine light.

Lotus: The blossom of the lotus plant, which grows in mud, is a symbol of beauty and spiritual completeness in the East, indicating that while the enlightened person lives in the mud of the material world, this in no way affects his true Self in his union with God . Light and harmony radiate out of such people, spreading love, joy and knowledge to the world. The scent of the lotus flower bears the same message, guiding the receptive and ready soul on its path to unity with God.

Understanding
the Astrological Associations

In esoteric publications a large variety of planets and signs of the zodiac are assigned to each chakra. Obviously, there are various systems, and each starts out at another point. There are, for instance, certain colors assigned to the planets and signs of the zodiac. From the characteristics associated with these colors we can draw conclusions about the corresponding chakras, which in turn also radiate in certain colors. Other systems are based on the elements assigned to both the signs of the zodiac and the chakras, while the relationships between organ systems and parts of the body also provide means of interpretation. Finally, there is also a method which establishes relationships between the seven chakras and the seven planets of classical astrology (Sun, Moon, Mercury, Venus, Mars, Jupiter and Saturn), whereby these planets are replaceable in part by the trans-Saturnial planets Uranus, Neptune and Pluto, which were discovered in relatively recent times and thus, with their characteristics, reflect the steps made forward in man's development.

As we see it, each of these astrological systems is of validity and recognizes various aspects of each chakra. In the chapters on the individual energy centers, we therefore mentioned the planets and signs of the zodiac that seem both logical and meaningful to us with regard to a better understanding of the chakras, along with a brief outline of their associated characteristics.

Possibilities for Cleansing and Activating the Chakras

Opening the chakras is a journey towards the Self, a journey into life and towards God. It is a holistic way of unfolding all the potential that you have as a human being.

The possibilities described here are sometimes called "therapy", although that does not mean to say that their application should be limited to therapeutic practice. The word "therapy" is derived from the Greek word "therapeia" which literally means "assisting someone on his way". In this sense, for instance, perfumes, sounds, colors and gemstones can also help us open and harmonize the chakras.

The positive effects of chakra therapy, however, will only be of duration when they accompany a process of growth and maturation. In order to achieve this, it is advisable to consider the following:

1. Choose one or more of the chakra therapies that appeal to you most and begin to practise them as regularly as possible. You will soon find out which individual measures are indispensable for your continuous development.

2. When the blockages in your chakras begin to dissolve, you may relive the experiences or feelings which caused them in the first place. Chronic illnesses can also enter an acute phase of temporary nature, similar to the reaction hoped for in certain forms of natural healing.

Let all these reactions happen without intervening or judging them. Suppress neither laughter nor tears, for everything you experience is a necessary and valuable aspect of the natural cleansing of your chakras. You will know yourself when such a cleansing process becomes too intense. In this case, let the measure in process come to a gentle end, remain still for a while and pay attention to the processes going on in your body and soul until they no longer oppress you.

3. Pay particular attention to the opening and harmonizing of your heart chakra, the center of the entire chakra system. This is the seat of the love which opens us to life and other people, a love capable of neutralizing all the tensions or blockages which could close your chakras again. By opening the heart chakra you ensure that the other chakras remain open and capable of expressing their potential in the best possible way.

4. Be sure to integrate all the experiences that come to you through the gradual opening of the chakras into everyday life. Do not reject anything,

but look at things in an open and loving way. Only by proceeding like this will you be able to understand what you experience and utilize it for your daily life and inner development.

Before we discuss the individual forms of therapy in greater detail, we would like to point out something which is fundamental for their understanding. Creation basically consists of pure, infinite consciousness, consisting of energy not yet manifest and without form or feature. When this consciousness begins to vibrate, energy structures come into being which bring forth the entire spectrum of life depending on wavelength, changes and transformation. The denser the vibrations of this primordial energy of consciousness are, the more they express themselves in a concrete and perceivable manner, devolving in the final analysis into what we call matter.

This principle is also known in quantum physics, which postulates a standardized field, a sphere consisting of the lowest stimulation of matter. It is this field which contains all stimulated states of matter in their latent form and it is from this field that they emerge to create the visible world. In the process during which this fundamental energy of consciousness becomes manifest, a number of basic vibrational patterns develop which permeate Creation at all levels.

As we know, colorless white light consists of the seven spectral colors which go to make up in turn the multitude of colours known on this world. The same basic vibrational patterns that manifest as colors in the sphere of light are also to be found in the realm of sound. Here, for example, a basic tone scale constitutes the foundation for an endless variety of musical works. The same applies to the abstract realm of numbers, the realm of form and movement (as expressed in dancing, for instance), and flora and fauna. It also holds true for the realm of fragrances, crystals, minerals and metals. Astrology expresses these basic patterns of vibration in the principles embodied by the individual planets and signs of the zodiac. In human beings these vibrations manifest in the form of characteristics, ideas and sensations, and in the functions of certain organ systems or parts of the body, which in turn correspond to various chakras. Thus, by applying the law of vibrational resonance, it is possible to influence the chakras. By merging our inner and outer senses with a particular vibrational pattern, we can revitalize and stimulate the vibration of the corresponding chakra.

We would like to illustrate this with an example. The influence of soft pink calls forth a sensation of gentleness and tender love in the heart chakra. On the plane of gemstones, rose quartz will produce a similar resonance, and on the level of music the gentle song of the harp or a violin will do the same. A tender, loving touch can also create a corresponding vibration in your heart chakra, thereby helping it to open and become active at its own vibrational level. According to this principle, you will find forms of expression corresponding to the principle of gentleness and tender love in all areas of Creation, and can thus awaken this principle within yourself on all levels of your being.

In the preceding chapters we have described the nature experiences, colors, gemstones, sounds and aromas that are helpful for treating the chakras. The clearer, purer and more natural the means you employ, the more effectively they will stimulate the vibration of your chakra in its pure, original form, thus neutralizing negative vibrations and disharmony.

Experiencing Nature

Nature offers an abundance of possibilities for cleansing, harmonizing and stimulating the chakras. The beauty of landscapes, bodies of waters, animals, plants and flowers corresponds to the vibration of the three lower chakras and strengthens and supports them in their functions. Together with the three higher chakras, the beauty of our planet helps the expression and stabilization of the energies of these chakras in the Here and Now. The sky, continually changing in light and color lit up by the stars at night, has an expanding and elevating influence on the three lower chakras and enhances the functions of the three higher chakras. The specific vibrations of the beauty of heaven and earth united into love in the heart chakra.

When you experience nature, it is good to do so in a mood of inner calmness, openness and gratitude. This will make you receptive for all kinds of healing, expanding and life-supporting influences.

As you become aware of the effect a particular nature experience is having on the corresponding chakra, gently direct your attention to it and surrender to all the sensations or feelings that may arise within you. They are an expression of the purifying and stimulating effect that nature is having on the chakra in question.

Sound Therapy

Sound consists of audible vibrations. If our hearing were to possess the necessary sensitivity to perceive all ranges of frequencies, we would be able to hear the music of flowers and grass, mountains and valleys, the singing of the sky and the stars and the symphony of our own body.

Modern science has confirmed what the mystics and wise men of old cultures knew and applied as a means of harmonizing, healing and expanding human consciousness: namely, that life basically consists of sound. It brought forth man and life on earth and maintains them in their existence.

Scientific findings confirm that all the particles in the universe, all forms of radiation, all natural forces and all information are determined by musical structures, frequencies and patterns and the high tones of their specific vibrations.

Indeed, from the billions of possible vibrations, the universe picks out the few thousand (with the surprising ratio of 1 : 1,000,000) that possess a harmonious character. These vibrations are expressed in the proportions of the overtones, certain ecclesiastical scales, the ragas of India, the major scale and, to a lesser extent, the minor scale.

The protons and neutrons of the oxygen atom, for instance, vibrate on a minor scale. When chlorophyll develops out of light and matter, triads ring out, and each flower and each blade of grass sings its own melody, their songs joining to form a harmonious whole. If this were not the case, they would not be able to thrive in each other's company, as proved by certain varieties of plants that avoid growing together.

We owe a great deal of our knowledge about plants to photo-acoustic spectroscopy, which, among other things, has made it possible to hear the blossoming of a rose bud. This sounds like an organ-like roar, very similar to a Bach toccata. Modern radio telescopy has also proven that the universe is full of sound, and that each celestial body has its own melody. The music we listen to is a reproduction of this music of life. In the religious ceremonies of many peoples it represents an expression of Creation itself. Music is a vital energy which penetrates all forms of manifestation, an energy strong enough to maintain and renew life. We can use it to attain unity with the life forces working in the innermost core of all things, thus bringing our energies into harmony with the life in the universe.

Not every kind of music is appropriate for this purpose. We all know that different kinds of music can evoke different feelings in us. Music can have a calming and relaxing effect and bring about a state of balance and harmony, it can stimulate, inspire and move us, or it can be simply superficial or trivial. Disharmonious sounds may cause nervousness, aggression and feelings of helplessness or discouragement.

The effects that different types of music can have been proved, among other means, in numerous experiments involving animals and plants. Hens, for instance, lay more eggs and cows yield more milk under the influence of classical music, while rock music produces a rapid decline in yield. Plants exposed to a constant barrage of rock music grow away from the speakers and gradually die, whereas when exposed to classical music they develop more rapidly and produce more leaves and flowers than plants exposed to no music at all. Moreover, plants apparently prefer the music of Bach, and in an experiment some inclined towards the speakers at an angle of 35°. Indian sitar music seems to have an even more positive influence, achieving growth angles of 60°. Indeed, in one experiment the nearest plants seemed to "embrace" the speakers, as if wanting to unite with this source of life-giving music. Country and folk music, on the other hand, seems to have no influence at all; plants react with indifference and their development and behavior does not differ in any way from plants not exposed to musical stimuli.

What holds true for plants and animals can also applied to human beings. If we want to activate and harmonize our energy centers with the help of music, we should select the music we listen to carefully.

The chapters about the individual chakras provide fundamental information about the forms of music suitable for the stimulation and harmonization of each energy center, but apart from our suggestions, you should also follow your own feelings in this matter. Take a look at your own collection of records and cassettes. Most likely you have some pieces suitable for chakra therapy, and you may already have a preference for the kind of music that stimulates a given chakra. Jot down the names of works that you like when they occur to you, and when you buy new cassettes or records, take into consideration which chakras the music will appeal to. You can also record three to five minute segments of your favorite music and thus create your own musical chakra tour. Let the individual sections begin and end softly. Tape the music for the root chakra first, and follow the sequence of the chakras accordingly.

Such a journey through the chakras awaits you on the cassette "Chakra Meditation"*, especially composed for chakra therapy and chakra medi-

---

*)"Chakra Meditation" by Shalila Sharamon and Bodo J. Baginski, Lotus Light Publications, Wilmot 1991

tation. Side one of this cassette serves as background music for the inner journey described at the end of this book, and side two consists of chakra music based on the knowledge that specific tones and keys are assigned to each energy center:

> the deep C and C major for the first chakra,
> D and D major for the second chakra,
> E and E major for the third chakra,
> F and F major for the fourth chakra,
> G and G major for the fifth chakra,
> A and A major for the sixth chakra, and
> H and H major for the seventh chakra

This music has been composed with instruments, rhythms and tonal sequences attuned to each individual chakra, and thus provides an optimal means of stimulating and harmonizing your energy centers and thus your entire being. This journey through the world of sound can be undertaken alone or used to support and augment the other forms of therapy described in this book.

Also well suited for this purpose is the "Spectrum Suite" composed by Steven Halpern in the keys assigned to each chakra. Like many other pieces of New Age music, it has been deliberately kept simple in character and has to be listened to in a new and "pure" manner free of the intellectual and emotional judgements we are used to applying.

As far as we know, the most extensive work of chakra music is the "Chakra Organ"*, published by Windpferd Verlag. It consists of seven separate sets, each containing a guide to chakra meditation, a cassette with chakra music (especially attuned to the corresponding energy center) and spoken meditation instructions. Each set also contains a special scent or mixture of scents and a specially selected gemstone. The cassettes themselves consist of a 60 minute program, comprising 30 minutes of chakra music and another 30 minutes of music with meditation instructions.

When you do chakra therapy, lie or sit down comfortably in a relaxed way. Should you be sitting, take care to maintain a straight back in order to let the energy flow between the individual chakras without hindrance.

Now open yourself to the sound of the music, let it flow into your body

---

*)"Chakra-Organ" by Marianne Uhl, Windpferd Verlag, D-8955 Aitrang, Germany, 1989

and soul. Allow its frequencies to transform the vibrations of mind, body and soul. Put all your ideas and expectations aside and enter the sound until you become one with it. During the first part of the music, direct your attention gently and effortlessly towards the root chakra and "see" what is happening there. Allow all the images and feelings the music awakens to rise within you. You will experience how the gradual ascent from one chakra to the next relaxes you more and more. At the same time, you will feel more alive and happier with every step you take. You may gain the impression that the music is affecting a particular center more intensely than others, or you may realize that some of the chakras are blocked. In this case you can stimulate the flow of energy in the chakra in question with crystals the next time you carry out chakra meditation. (In this respect, please see the chapter on gemstone therapy.)

When the music fades away, enjoy the silence for a while. It is a living silence, a silence that you have probably rarely experienced. Just as colorless light contains all the colors of the spectrum, this silence contains all the sounds of the universe. It awakens your soul and makes it receptive for the Divine sound that permeates all manifestation and the messages it reveals. Imagine this silence flowing into your energy centers, beginning with the crown chakra.

You can repeat this purifying and stimulating "bath" in spiritual energy every morning and evening - or whenever you feel like it.

If you have a favorite piece of music that calms and relaxes you, while expanding your consciousness and filling you with joy, you can certainly utilize it as background music for any form of therapy.

We also want to recommend dancing. Once you have arranged your musical journey through the chakras, dance to its music whenever you feel like it. Let your body find its own forms of expression. This dancing lets you join in the vital moving dance of creation on all levels. The energies of these levels find expression through your body and thus have an influence on your daily life. Of course, you can also dance to the music of individual chakras if your main intention is to unite with and actively express the power of this particular energy center.

There are also two very effective forms of sound therapy or meditations which utilize the voice. The vibrations thus generated permeate you on the inside and the outside. Moreover, you only need to intone one single note to stimulate each individual chakra.

As we know from the teachings on overtones, every single tone contains all others, even if we are unable to perceive this. When one string resounds - and our vocal chords correspond to the strings of an instrument - it is not only the whole string (or the fundamental tone) that is vibrating, but also half of the string, or the next higher octave. And so it goes on: not only the whole and half string vibrate, but also two-thirds, or a quinte; also three-quarters, or a fourth; three-fifths, or a major sext; four-fifths, or a major third; and five-sixths, or a minor third. This means that the entire scale vibrates in sympathy as an overtone series. In India there are various instruments which specially emphasize and stress the overtones, making them audible for the human ear. Something similar occurs in overtone singing.

The fact that overtones occur when a certain note is played is of interest in that each tone we sing to stimulate a certain energy center automatically affects the other chakras, meaning that by stimulating one chakra, all are stimulated.

You can practise both these forms of sound therapy standing or sitting - preferably in the lotus or cross-legged position - or else with your bottom between your heels in the diamond position.

The first form of sound therapy uses the notes assigned to the chakras as well as vowel sounds. Here we have to remember that 'm' is considered a vowel in India. The effects that the different vowels have are described in the chapters on the individual chakras.

Sing the vowels when you exhale. Do this three times at normal volume, all the while directing your attention towards the corresponding chakra until you feel the note vibrating in this sphere.

Starting out with the root chakra, sing the vowels in the following order:

	'u' (ooh) in deep C for the first chakra
a closed	'o' in D for the second chakra
an open	'o' in E for the third chakra
	'ah' in F for the fourth chakra
	'eh' in G for the fifth chakra
	'e' in A for the sixth chakra
	'm' in H for the seventh chakra.

The entire cosmos is contained in these vowel sounds. They lead you into all spheres and are crowned by the 'm' of everlasting unity.

You can now ascend and descend the tones again. When you have finished, sit a while in silence, as described earlier, and let your feelings slowly resonate to an end.

The second form of sound therapy using the voice consists of using the root mantras assigned to the chakras instead of vowels. Mantras are syllables of meditation, so to speak, that work on a vibrational level. They express certain aspects of the individual Divine unity and connect the devotee with cosmic energy. In chakra meditation we use the so-called *Bija* or root mantras. *Bija* means energy, seed, or cosmic energy beyond all material manifestation. Here, the expression of highest unity is greatly concentrated. We would like to list the Bija mantras that stimulate the individual chakras again:

> LAM for the first chakra
> VAM for the second chakra
> RAM for the third chakra
> YAM for the fourth chakra
> HAM for the fifth chakra
> KSHAM for the sixth chakra
> OM for the seventh chakra.

As far as we know, the traditional teachings do not mention singing or intoning the root mantras to certain notes. We believe, however, that you should determine yourself whatever you find most pleasant and effective. If you wish, you can also recite the mantras to yourself without making audible sound whatsoever.

Considering how little time is required, you will probably find it easy to practise the last two forms of sound therapy or meditation every day. As in all other forms of therapy, be sure to wear natural fabrics if possible, and surround yourself with natural materials. At the beginning of this chapter we described how all things create their own music. These vibrations have an influence on us, although to a lesser extent than the vibrations of audible music and perceptible sound. They produce a resonance within us that can change our own vibrational pattern or disturb its harmonious functioning. We assume that all naturally developed objects produce sounds which are in harmony and which therefore harmonize us with the great symphony of Creation. Artificial fabrics and materials, however, bring about disharmony in most cases, comparable with the unpleasant sounds made by machines. This may be a reason why sensitive people do not feel comfortable in a world of plastic or in clothes made of synthetics.

If you regularly practise one of these sound therapies, you will feel yourself opening up more and more to the music of life.

At the end of this chapter we would like to cite the following words by the Indian Sufi musician Hazrat Inayat Khan:

"We can find the experience of harmony and unity everywhere, in the beauty of nature, in the colors of the flowers, in everything we see and come across, in the hours of meditation and solitude as well as in the hours of active life in the midst of our world. Everywhere we perceive music and joyfully experience its harmony. By breaking down the walls surrounding us, we experience unity with the Absolute. This unity is a manifestation of the music of the spheres."

Color Therapy

Colors are sounds made visible. Their frequencies, however, are imperceptible for our ears. In order to let us perceive them, nature created another medium: our eyes. Colors exert a powerful influence on us through their specific vibrations (wavelengths or frequencies), regardless of whether we are conscious of this fact or not. We are constantly exposed to the influence of colors - starting out with the blue of the sea and the sky, the green of the woods and meadows, the brown of the earth and the yellow of desert sand and the changing kaleidoscope of the colors of the rising or setting sun. Our own individual environment is also influenced and shaped by the color of our clothes and bed linen, our furniture and wallpaper and even our food. Everywhere we are exposed to color vibrations and are consciously or unconsciously influenced by them.

It is therefore only logical and natural to put colors to conscious use. Color vibrations influence us through the seven chakras in a very special manner. In the previous chapters we described which color is closely related to which chakra. Essentially, one color of the spectrum is assigned to each energy center. We all know that when a ray of light falls onto a prism, it refracts into the seven colors of the rainbow. In nature these

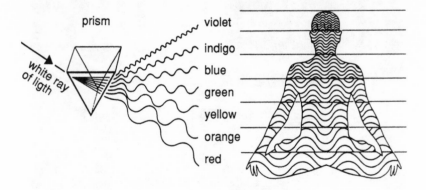

A white ray of light is broken into the seven colors of the spectrum by a prism, thus creating the different wavelengths or frequencies of these colors, shown here in accordance with their respective chakras.

colors become visible in a drop of dew or rain, and achieve their most perfect form in the rainbow, of course. Here we can contemplate the play of the spectral colors in their purest form of expression, and when we employ colors to heal, these should also be as pure as possible.

In our therapeutic practice we often use a special color therapy lamp*, into which colored glass plates can be inserted to provide our clients with the various color wavelengths. This rather simple measure has proven to be very effective, although a special color radiation unit beaming on all seven chakras simultaneously would be even more effective. However, such a device has not been constructed but it could be designed in the following manner:

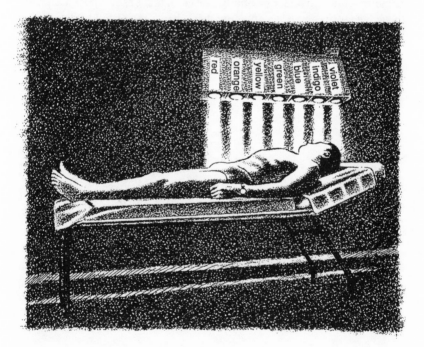

* For information on manufacturers and additional details, please see page 191

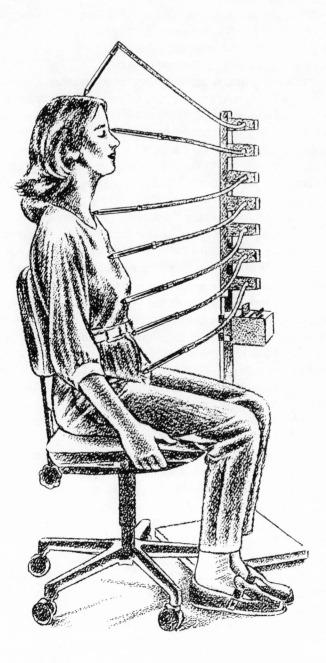

A gemstone beam unit

Of course you can also use a normal desk lamp with a filter of colored paper to treat each chakra or the entire body for five to ten minutes. (If you employ this method, be especially careful due to the fire hazard posed by the proximity of paper and a light bulb.)

Another very interesting possibility for color radiation treatment was developed several years ago by gemstone researcher Joachim Roller. He constructed special miniaturized spotlights that shine through various gemstones. The vibration of the bundled ray of light thus beamed through the gemstones is thus greatly improved. The individual gemstone spots can be easily adjusted to shine on a seated person. The principle of this particular form of treatment is based on knowledge of Ayurveda, which Joachim Roller studied thoroughly over a long period of time.

The therapeutic success of this method has been demonstrated in a number of symposiums and speaks for itself. The gemstone beam kits are available both individually and as a chakra set.

Knowledge of the special influence of filtered light is nothing new. Back in the ancient cultures of Greece and Egypt, colors were employed specifically and with great effect to heal the sick. Depending on the illness, the patients were brought into special rooms with windows covered by cloths dyed blue, red, violet, etc. In this manner the incoming light gained another quality that proved beneficial for certain physical and mental conditions. Of course, this method can also be employed today. The stained glass windows in churches also lend the incoming light another quality. We assume that the builders of the great churches and cathedrals of the past knew about the effect of color and consciously utilized it.

Obviously, the color of our clothes and even underwear has a considerable influence upon our well-being. If you want to activate a specific chakra, be sure that the clothing for this part of your body is of the right color. You can also influence your well-being with the color of your bedding. If you constantly feel weak and devoid of energy, red wallpaper, curtains and bunches of red flowers in your surroundings will help. The red color of food, drinks and spices can also be used to stimulate a weak first chakra. Beetroot, which is used to correct anaemia, is also appropriate in color therapy. There is no limit to what the imagination can come up with in color therapy - all you have to do is remember the basic principles of the chakra colors.

We should also keep in mind that all Creation is built up in accordance with certain logical color principles. It is not by coincidence that our blood is of the same color as the glow of fire or the interior of a volcano. Whenever we come upon the color red we are confronted with energy and activity. A radiant red rose attracting insects to pollinate it employs the same principle as a night club which seeks to stimulate thoughts of sex with red lighting. We are all familiar with the term "red light district" for the part of a city with lots of brothels. In the context of sexuality the color red expresses purely physical desire, whereas the color orange, which is assigned to the second chakra, invites us to enjoy a more refined form of sensuality which entails feelings of love and which makes us feel happy. It is interesting to note that for years the favorite color of Bhagwan's followers has been orange. These few examples prove that the influence of colors is recognized and employed to a certain extent in modern-day life, but nonetheless, this only applies to a few limited spheres. A simple and effective way of employing the beneficial effects of color is to know the colors assigned to the seven chakras and apply them according to the chakra teachings.

Who would want to fire up a volcano even more? In life, however, this happens frequently. A good example of this is an episode Bodo once experienced. One day a nun came to his practice complaining of problems in her lower back. As she lay on the examination table, Bodo was surprised to find her wearing bright red underwear. As it was barely conceivable that she could give free vent to her sexuality, a massive overload of energy had accumulated at the lower end of her spinal column (in the first chakra region). In this case, the particular color of the underwear was definitely inappropriate. If she had chosen a shade of violet, instead, it would have helped transform the overload into spiritual energy, while a blue color would have dampened or neutralized it.

An example such as this underlines the far-reaching implications of color vibrations. We have recounted this admittedly extraordinary experience because it is certainly not easy to forget the picture of a nun wearing bright red underpants.

When we are aware of the interaction between colors and our energy centers, we can employ color in a conscious and purposeful manner. If we want to activate the heart chakra, for instance, we should utilize soft pink colors as much as possible: we can decorate our home and place of work with pink flowers, wear pink clothes and put on the legendary rose-tinted glasses to see the world quite literally in this color. There are also rose-colored light bulbs, pink candles or even bath additives. And when we prepare ourselves a yoghurt or a pudding, why not choose a pink one? Our jewellery could consist of rose quartz or we could put some rose-colored gemstones on our night table, our desk and in the kitchen. Should you wish to surround yourself permanently with this soft color of the heart, you could decorate your home or at least one particular room in pink.

In our culture, pink is the favorite color for baby girls, and adult women often choose rose-colored underwear. Obviously, it is regarded as a very feminine characteristic to want to stimulate the subtle vibrations of love in the heart chakra. However, we would like to encourage men to put aside such conventions and surround themselves with rose-colored stimuli whenever appropriate.

In case there is no way to expose yourself to a particular color vibration, you should choose colorless white or white light, which, as already mentioned, contains the entire color spectrum and thus the specific color you need (white light means pure white light, not fluorescent light). When you wear white clothes or expose yourself to sunlight, you automatically utilize the entire color spectrum, too. The ancient Greek and Egyptians were aware of the beneficial effects of this phenomenon. During the daytime they would put the sick out in the sun or wrap them in white cloth.

Black has the opposite effect, as it possesses the lowest color vibration of all. It is therefore also the most unfavorable color treatment. Black clothing worn permanently leads to a considerable dampening of all chakra functions, and people with marked instability will notice these effects very soon.

Whenever we are faced with the decision of whether to act in harmony with nature or against her laws, the choice is ours. We are free - so let us decide!

Chakra Color Meditation

"By mind I understand that power of the soul which thinks and develops concepts."

(Aristotle, 384 - 322 B.C.)

All the measures described up to now are methods in which you open yourself up to an outside influence and allow yourself to be influenced by it. However, there are also excellent ways of treating yourself with colors in an inner way, although they require a little effort on your part. People who by their very nature like take an active part in shaping their destiny often consider such methods the most effective means of influencing the chakras in a positive way.

The magic word here is "visualization", or "guided imagination". Visualization is a natural capability that all human beings have and which is not difficult to practise. Today a great many doctors and psychologists use this procedure for the treatment of cancer, among other things, with great success. It concerns the creative ability to form a mentally visual images not present to the eye, and it is a highly interesting fact that our mind is capable of turning such mental images into reality. To achieve this, however, we have to completely affirm what we see and genuinely want to make it become true.

Most people learn the technique quite rapidly, while others need a bit of practise. In all cases the effort is certainly worthwhile.

In this context it is interesting to note that people with a strong fire sign influence (Aries, Leo or Sagittarius) generally have a distinct talent for visualization. As we know from the chakra teachings, the sensual function of vision is assigned to the fire element. People with a dominant earth sign influence (Taurus, Virgo or Capricorn) tend to find it more difficult. Since the sense of smell is assigned to the earth element, these people generally respond better to aroma therapy. In other words, there are areas in life where we feel instinctively at home, and areas that we first have to get used to. That's the way Mother Nature determined it, and there is certainly sense to it.

Everything we need for visualization we contain within us. We do not need any external assistance, just a bit of time. Since the chakras immediately react to inner images conjured up in this way, the visualization of colors is an excellent and effective means of influencing them positively.

Chakra color meditation can be practised standing, sitting or lying down. All that is important is that the spine should be completely straight. Once we are comfortable, we close our eyes and calm down. Our breathing is quiet and regular. Whenever thoughts arise we let them pass without paying attention to them. In this way we grant ourselves a few minutes of silence. We grow calmer and calmer and allow ourselves to be taken over by a feeling of inner stillness and security.

We now direct our attention towards the bottom of the pelvic girdle, the sphere of the first chakra, which opens downward. Here we visualize a small spark of red light. We let it get bigger and bigger until it becomes a ball of radiant red light. This may take a minute or longer. Time is irrelevant, the only thing that matters is the image we create - and the longer we manage to hold it, the more effective the exercise will be. Whenever the inner image begins to slip away, we visualize it in our mind's eye again, without any pressure or compulsive effort. The whole business is just a game - but it is a very special game, a game that plays with the primordial energies of the cosmos, the laws of manifestation.

Remain aware your limit. Know when it is time to stop. Two or three minutes of visualization will usually be quite enough, as we want to activate our chakras, not overload them. After having visualized the ball of fiery red light, shift your attention slowly and smoothly to your second chakra, a handbreadth below the navel. Visualize a spark of clear orange. Let it become bigger, brighter and clearer. Try to see the resulting ball of light as clearly and as long as possible. Do not expend any effort; the more natural the process, the better. When you feel you've had enough, move on to the next center. This is the solar plexus chakra, and is about two fingers above the navel. Imagine an impulse in a bright, golden light and let it grow. After holding your attention on it a few minutes, wander up to your heart chakra smoothly and effortlessly and imagine a spark that is pink at the center and green on the outside. Visualize it until you can see the colors clearly. Let them grow in size and enjoy their beauty for a while. A deep feeling of satisfaction will set in.

Now move on to the throat center and visualize a spark of bright blue. Don't push or press yourself, just follow your intuition. Don't overdo things - you should always feel at ease during this exercise.

Our journey of colors continues up to the bridge of the nose at the front of the forehead. Here we visualize a small stimulus of color in a deep indigo blue. The impulse grows and grows until it forms a splendid ball of color. Try to hold the image as long as possible in your mind's eye. The only thing that matters is this ball shining in indigo blue.

Now we come to the culmination of our exercise, to the crown chakra. Visualize a small spark of violet light developing at the center of your head, at the highest point. Let it grow into a violet flame with golden rays. Perhaps it is shinings more magnificently than the other chakras. What a wonderful and elevating feeling it is to be crowned by a halo of light! We let the rays spread out around us as far as they reach.

Now we are finished, we keep our eyes closed and remain in silence for a while. Altogether, this meditational exercise will take about 20 minutes. If you now listen within, you will notice that you are calm and balanced, yet full of inner strength, energy and joy. You are open, yet protected; you are centered within yourself but with your feet firmly on the ground. You realize that your spirit has opened and balanced your energy centers. You are the master not only of your physical body but also of your subtle ones. You have just experienced this in an unmistakable manner.

While we, Bodo and Shalila, were writing these lines, we visualized our own chakras, thus activating and harmonizing them in the process. Although it only took a few minutes, we feel as if we have been on a short vacation, and so we are doubly grateful for having explained this form of visualization to you. It is one of the most amazing ways of healing and harmonizing your body, soul and spirit yourself. As a rule it requires less time than a trip to the drugstore, and it is completely natural, meaning that you can do it twice a day if you want to. Of course you can combine this visualization exercise with other forms of chakra therapy, such as sound therapy, aroma therapy, breathing exercises, etc.

Please do not try to understand this form of meditation on an intellectual level alone, for that would be of little benefit to you. It is your personal experience, your inner knowledge will take you further along the path - especially with the help of this wonderful and simple method. Your power lies in the Here and Now, in your consciousness. Try it out - the effort is worth while!

Gemstone Therapy

All the advanced forms of civilization we know of appreciated gemstones not only for their beauty but also for their healing and harmonizing powers. They have grown through millions of years in the bowels of the earth, experiencing a process of refinement, cleansing and purification in darkness and seclusion before being discovered by Man in their most perfect form and brought to the light of the world.

Gemstones are suited for chakra therapy in a very special way. Created out of the elements of our Mother Earth, they connect us with the protecting, fortifying and nourishing energy of this earth. They bear light in its purest and most natural colors and transmit cosmic characteristics and energy. They attract and channel the forces of both the sky and earth and radiate them out into the world. Their crystalline structure reflects principles of order that establish contact between us and the cosmic order as well as having a harmonizing influence on body and soul.

When you carry a gemstone on your person, a fine resonance of vibrations sets up within you. All the inner powers and characteristics within you which are blocked, buried or distorted will answer to the vibrations of the gemstones and thus be awakened and revived to their original form.

You should always use gemstones of the very best quality for chakra therapy. The clearer the stone and the purer its structure, the clearer and purer will be the energy it radiates and activates within you.

Before using gemstones you should cleanse them, as they do not only transmit energy but also absorb harmful substances from the body and negative vibrations from the ethereal body and the environment, thus purifying and protecting you. Some stones, however, may become discolored or cracked in cleansing and should no longer be used. If this happens, return them to the earth. After a while, you can dig them out again and see if they have recovered their original color and clarity.

In order to cleanse gemstones you can use water and sea salt. For a short cleansing it is sufficient to wash them one or two minutes under running water and dry them afterwards with a clean cloth made of natural fibre. The cleaning vibrations of water carry away everything negative the stones have taken on.

Should you wish a more thorough cleansing, leave the stones under running water for several hours. Most appropriate would be a stream with natural clear water, but if absolutely necessary, tap water will also do.

Another possibility is to put the gemstones in water with natural sea salt over night, or to keep them in dry sea salt. In this case they should be completely covered by the salt, which should not be used again afterwards. It would be best if you also gave it back to the purifying force of the earth. After cleansing you can load the stones with energy by exposing them to sunlight for a few hours.

If your gemstones are used frequently, they should be cleansed and reloaded with energy from time to time. In most cases you will get to know when it is time again to cleanse them. If you use them during an illness, it is advisable to wash them under running water each time you use them.

Whenever you buy gemstones or receive them as gifts they have probably made a long journey and absorbed all kinds of unknown vibrations in the process. Therefore, you should cleanse them thoroughly and, if possible, load them with sunlight before using them the first time. They will then be able to transmit their energies to you in the best possible way.

As described in the chapters on the various chakras, several gemstones are assigned to each energy center. If you want to carry out gemstone therapy on your chakras, choose a stone with the specific properties which seem most useful to you at the moment. You can also let yourself be guided by your intuition and choose a stone which attracts you in a special way as you might not always be aware of the energy you need the most. Naturally, you can also use stones which have not been described here.

To treat your chakras with gemstones, make sure that you will not be interrupted for about half an hour and choose a place where you can lie down comfortably. (You can also enhance the treatment with music and fragrances, as described in the respective chapters.) Lie down on your back and stretch out your legs.

Put the gemstone on the individual chakras. Best results are achieved when you place them on the skin. Lay the stone for the root chakra in your crotch, between the anal outlet and the genitals, where closefitting underpants will easily hold it in place. The stone you have chosen for the sacral chakra should be placed at the upper edge of the pubic hair.

Now place the stone for the solar plexus center approximately two fingerbreadths above the navel. The gemstone which corresponds to the heart chakra should be laid in the middle of your chest at the height of the heart. If you like, you can also use two stones here, a green one and a pink one. You can also use two stones for the throat chakra if you want. The first one should be placed on the pit of your throat and the second under your neck, at the nape. Put the stone for the inner eye above the bridge of the nose between your brows, and place the gemstone for the crown chakra at the top your head. If the stone has a natural tip, point this in the direction of your head.

As soon as all the gemstones are in place, return your arms to your sides, close your eyes and contemplate how the energies are flowing within you. Since gemstones act of their accord, it is not necessary to visualize what is going on or repeat affirmations. Forget what you expect to happen and trust that everything now happening has to happen to lead you to inner wholeness. Do not analyze or evaluate what you are experiencing. The energy of the stones is awakening the natural self-healing power within you which knows of itself how to bring you back to a state of wholeness again. Trust in its guidance and accept the reactions and the processes of healing, purification and awareness that are taking place within you. Do not dispel or suppress what you feel, but do not make them happen either. Your limited understanding, which is full of value judgements, cannot compete with natural healing energy. It alone will find the best way.

If you have the feeling that a particular chakra needs more energy or thorough cleansing and harmonization, you can support the action of the particular gemstone by pointing some rock crystals around the stone. You can reinforce the energies of several chakras at the same time in this way. Another way to intensify the effect of a gemstone is to hold a rock crystal in each hand, thus incorporating the hand chakras. Point the crystal in your right hand away from your arm and the crystal in your left hand towards it, thus creating a continual circle of energy in which the right hand radiates energy and the left receives it.

You can have a wonderfully deep and intense gemstone experience with at least six rock crystals and some black tourmaline sticks. Black tourmalines are like lightning rods for negative energy. Lie down and place the rock crystals around your body (the points should be towards you), the first about 10 cm above your head. Put one or two more below your feet and the rest to the right and left of your body. Now lay the tourmaline sticks between the rock crystals. If the sticks come to a natural end, this should be turned away from your body.

You are now surrounded by a circle of radiant rock crystal light. Negative vibrations from your environment are kept away; At the same time, negative vibrations are led away from you aura. Lying in such a protective, revitalizing and purifying circle of light is a wonderful and profound experience. As it may turn out to be very intense, you should not undergo this form of gemstone therapy too frequently.

Another form of gemstone treatment consists of using rock crystals alone for all the chakras, since the pure white light of the rock crystal contains the energy potential of all seven colors of the rainbow, which in turn correspond to the seven chakras. For this reason, a rock crystal will stimulate all the chakras and harmonize the entire energy system.

You can also position the rock crystals in such a way that they point towards your heart. As for the heart chakra itself, place one rock crystal here pointing towards your head and the other towards your feet. In this way all the energy flows towards the center of the chakra system, our heart, from where it is radiated out again. This is only one way of positioning the crystals. Feel free to try out other systems, if you wish. You can also employ polished or cut rock crystals.

As a rule, gemstone therapy should not exceed 20 minutes in length, and sometimes even five minutes will be sufficient. After you remove the stones from your body, it is advisable to remain lying down with your eyes closed for a few minutes to let the experience reverberate within you. Of course, you can also make the vibrations of gemstones part of your everyday life by wearing them as jewelry or carrying them in your pocket. To this end choose one or more stones with properties you consider desirable. Sometimes such a gemstone will become a constant companion. You may also want to position one or more gemstones in a place where you spend a lot of time.

We already briefly discussed another, very special form of gemstone therapy in the chapter about color therapy: the use of gemstone beam units. Joachim Roller*, the gemstone researcher mentioned in that

* For information on manufacturers and additional details, please see page 191

chapter, has also developed a special gemstone balm containing genuine gemstone powder for each chakra. It is applied to the area of the respective chakra and has a healing, revitalizing and protecting effect.

Finally, we would like to give you some general advice about handling gemstones. The outer form of a gemstone is sustained by an inner being. Remember that whenever you direct your loving attention on a being, you open yourself to the gifts it has to give you. This is not only true for human beings but also for animals, plants and minerals. Therefore, you should treat stones with love and respect, appreciate their gifts and store them in a place where they will delight your eyes and heart again and again.

Aroma Therapy

All plants, animals and human beings possess a distinct, individual odor, although it sometimes requires a highly developed sense of smell to perceive and distinguish it in each case. Our odor expresses our personality, our individual characteristics and the state of our health. We usually associate a pleasant odor with health, vitality and harmony. A healthy newborn baby radiates a subtle, wonderfully sweet scent similar to that of ripe peaches. People who have managed to completely cleanse their bodies by repeated fasting, healthy diet and meditation exude a comparable fragrance.

Whenever we smell anything pleasant, we automatically inhale deeply and fill our lungs with the aromatic, life-giving scent that has such a stimulating and life-giving effect on us. When we come across an unpleasant smell, we instinctively hold our breath to prevent something unhealthy and wrong from entering us, something not beneficial to life. What we perceive as pleasant or unpleasant is totally dependent on past experience and our way of life. A smoker, for instance, probably has a positive but totally different impression of the smell of cigarette smoke than someone who detests smoking and is be nauseated by the same smell.

It has been customary throughout history to burn incense in the presence of kings, priests and sacred objects. Perhaps the earliest form of aroma therapy, the burning of incense was also carried out as protection against the plague and other diseases. Especially distinctive scents were employed to drive away evil spirits, evoke the favor of the gods or attune people to the higher spheres. The ancient Greeks, Egyptians, Babylonians, Indians and Chinese, to mention only a few cultures, used fragrant essences to correct states of imbalance, harmonize energy, heal and prevent illnesses, cleanse and purify, bring about relaxation and stimulate.

As in the case of many other methods of natural healing, the use of aromas has been rediscovered as a form of therapy and is now the subject of a great deal of interest.

The essential beings of plants, each with its own individual characteristics and message, seeks to serve us - with their colors, their active substances and their fragrances - to enhance our health, provide us with joy and expand consciousness. By extending their roots deep into the earth and their leaves up towards the light, they take in earthly and celestial energies which they then transform into beauty, color and scent before passing them on to us. The aromatic essences of plants consist of their innermost being in unspoiled purity, prepared to radiate out generously when the proper moment is at hand. Their fragrant scents combine with the energies of the soul and bring about processes of transformation within us.

You may have already experienced for yourself how the scent of a joss stick or an aroma lamp can enhance the atmosphere of a room, creating a "climate" that both relaxes us and lightens our burdens. We see things more clearly and our spirit becomes more lucid. We feel the subtle, bright substance of our soul remembering that it has wings, that the heaviness and gloom of bothersome problems does not belong to its true being and that it is free and capable of rising above time and space. With the help of fragrant essences we really can leave troubles behind or learn to view them more objectively and from a new perspective. A clear and light-hearted feeling of joy will spread through us as we perceive things on a finer level and experience time without pressure or haste.

Recent investigations have shown that scents make the most intense impression of all on the senses and that they have a direct influence our state of mind.

No other sensual function reaches the information stored within our unconscious as directly as the sense of smell. At some time in your life you have doubtlessly smelled a certain odor, and were immediately swept back into another time and place, and relived the feelings connected with this smell. Usually the memories that come to us like this are most enjoyable ones. The fact of the matter is that these ethereal substances act at a very deep and fundamental level of our being, in a sphere that lies far beyond our blocked energies and unresolved problems, in an area of the soul where we are very close to pure Being, as proved by the memories of spontaneous joy that pleasant fragrances so often trigger off. Essential oils are capable of leading us to these levels of well-being while dissolving the blockages that would otherwise stand in our way.

The subtle ethereal substances of flowers and plants touch the energy body of human beings, the seat of the chakras, and unfold their healing, harmonizing energies.

Be sure to use only the purest plant essences when you carry out aroma therapy for the chakras, as all artificially produced scents lack the vital energy of the plants as well as the complex mixture of ingredients that only Mother Nature is capable of combining. The users of modern, synthetic scents and perfumes have no part in the exquisite world of natural fragrances and their powers.

Since these essences are of natural origin, their effects are in perfect harmony with the necessities of your body and soul. They often also have a normalizing effect; that is, they tend to bring about a condition of healthy, harmonious well-being.

Fragrant essences are here on earth to be smelled, for it is this which enables them to release their active ingredients. These ingredients are not transmitted alone by inhalation, however. The essences also radiate vibrations which do not require the nose as a medium at all, but which have a direct influence on us. It was once observed, for example, that a female peacock butterfly attracted dozens of males against the wind from over a distance of miles, thus proving that they were not attracted by her scent.

When we activate our chakras with the help of essential oils, we benefit from both the ways they have of transmitting their qualities. The effects of various scents and the chakras they are associated with have been described in detail in the preceding chapters. Be sure to use a different fragrance for each chakra. And please remember that our list is meant as a suggestion, not as a set of rules. For example, all sweet-smelling flower oils have an especially harmonizing influence on the sacral chakra, although they are recommended for all chakras. Lavender is also suitable for relaxing the inner eye chakra, while rosemary has a stimulating influence on the root chakra. It is best if you follow both the feelings scents awaken in you and your intuition when following our suggestions.

Aroma therapy is well-suited for implementation in combination with color visualization and the various forms of sound and gemstone therapy, but is best combined with the breathing exercises described further back. Our breath serves as a medium for the interchange of energies between scents and chakras when we deeply inhale the vibrations of essential oils. If you want to apply the oils directly to your skin, it is advisable to mix them in a 10% solution with vegetable oils (jojoba, almond or sesame oil, etc.), or to put two drops of the undiluted essence onto a cotton ball which you then place on the chakra. We recommend preparing the cotton balls ahead of time and placing them nearby. Begin treatment with the root chakra and do not apply the next essential oil until your consciousness has shifted to the chakra about to be treated. A few minutes per chakra are generally sufficient. In other therapy forms (excluding aroma therapy), you can add an aromatic touch by lighting joss sticks or an aroma lamp. And now, let the fragrances take over, lift you up and carry you away into new spheres of consciousness.

Forms of Yoga

When people of the Western Hemisphere hear the word "Yoga", they frequently associate it with the physical exercises of Hatha Yoga, which can be fairly complicated. However, this is only one form of Yoga, and the true significance of Yoga as a whole goes far beyond carrying out exercises for health. Literally translated, Yoga means "yoke", which implies harnessing oneself to the Divine with the intention of uniting with it. Every way leading to such a union can be called Yoga, and all forms can be undertaken at various levels. In this sense the term Yoga apples to most forms of meditation.

In the chapters on the individual chakras one or more form of Yoga have been assigned to each energy center. They revitalize the chakra in question in a special way, namely by achieving the union that all forms of Yoga strive for.

If you wish to practise Yoga or meditation, the forms we have suggested for each chakra may be of help. What we cannot do within the framework of this book, however, is analyze each of the different possibilities in detail. Besides, many of the forms of Yoga mentioned here should be learned from a qualified teacher if their full potential is to be attained. All of them are highly effective ways of purifying and harmonizing the entire chakra system.

Chakra Breathing

Perhaps at some point in your life you have already become aware of the fact that breathing connects you with everything that surrounds you. Human beings, animals and plants all breathe the same air. You inhale the air they have exhaled, and vice versa. Our breathing not only unites us with the external world, it also establishes continuous contact and exchange with the internal world. Our breath reaches the tiniest and most distant cells and supplies our body with vital energy.

From Sanskrit writings we know of the term *prana*, which has been translated as respiration, breath or universal cosmic energy. These varying translations describe the different levels of breathing. Through breathing we are in fact in contact with the all-permeating life force, without which there would be no Creation as we know it. Here we become conscious of the dimensions of respiration, a process which is taken for granted yet which is of universal significance.

Therefore it is not surprising that practically all spiritually advanced cultures attach special importance to breathing and have based a large variety of consciousness-expanding exercises on this fact. The Eastern traditions regard breathing as more than the simple process of respiration, however. Although people all over the world basically inhale the same gaseous mixture, the way it is breathed in is the deciding factor. Breathing carried out in a certain set and conscious way obviously enhances the healing and harmonizing effects of the vital energy contained in the air. One could go so far as to say that through consciousness we unlock and benefit from certain energy frequencies in the air. In accordance, subtly graded breathing techniques have been developed over the ages, and are highly esteemed in practically all spiritual and health-conscious circles. When we deliberately direct our consciousness to our breathing, we can bring about enormously positive effects. The influence that breathing can have on the chakras also has a long tradition, so it is understandable that many special techniques have also been developed in this area. We would now like to describe a simple chakra breathing method which is highly effective and which can be practised at home by anyone.

We lie down or seat ourselves comfortably while maintaining a straight back. After a few moments of stillness we begin to breathe calmly and regularly, preferably through the nose. Then we imagine that as we inhale and exhale, we are drawing the air in and releasing it through our chakras. We begin this by directing our attention to the root chakra and imagining that we are breathing through it gently and slowly. We let the revitalizing *prana* stream flow in at its ease, and let if flow out again equally unhurriedly. We continue this for about 3 to 5 minutes, and then move on to the next energy center, the sacral chakra, and breathe through it in the same manner. And thus we continue, moving on to the next center every 3 to 5 minutes until we have reached the crown chakra. It is important that our consciousness always stays with the chakra we are breathing through and is not allowed to drift away.

Practically everyone who has done this simple exercise feels harmonious and balanced and yet full of energy afterwards. Some are completely overwhelmed, and we've often heard comments like, "I feel reborn", "I'm a new person", or "I really feel rejuvenated." A few people have the feeling of finally being centered, while others simply feel calm and relaxed.

It is really wonderful what such a simple exercise can bring about! It is truly a source of joy, peace, power and love, and is highly effective, especially for people suffering from depression or feeling weak and drained. Through chakra breathing we can recharge our energy system with properly aligned power.

Another possibility consists of combining chakra breathing with the vibrations of gemstones, fragrances, sounds and colors. While applying the methods described in the previous chapters, simply consciously breathe in their energies through the chakras. This method is also highly effective.

You may also wish to try out dynamic chakra breathing. Here you do not breathe gently, but use your imagination to breathe forcefully and rapidly through your chakras. This method has in fact been labelled "Chakra Breathing"* and is very popular among the followers of Bhagwan Shree Rajneesh. The spoken instructions are available on cassette, which we definitely recommend, as the written word does not really suffice to describe the effects of dynamic chakra breathing. It must be said, however, that while this particularly energetic form of breathing ignites a tremendous "fire" within the person practising it, it requires effort and hard work. For some it can became **the** method for cleansing and activating their chakras, while others do not feel all that enthusiastic about it at all. In this, as in all cases, simply follow your inner voice, which will always guide you to what is best for you.

Some of you will have probably already heard about *pranayama* or tried the techniques connected with it. The word *pranayama* is Sanskrit andmeans "mastery of *prana*". The breathing techniques involved stimu-

---

*Available as a cassette (labelled "Chakra Breathing") from all Rajneesh centers.

late and harmonize the energy potential of the chakras, but should be learned under the personal guidance of a qualified teacher, if possible. No matter which method we apply, the effort is always worthwhile.

Chakra Reflex Zone Massage

For many of us it is a long established fact that every part of the body and every organ system has its corresponding reflex zone. The best-known reflex zones are those of the feet, where the entire organism is represented in small areas or zones. As these reflex zones are in close reflective connection with their corresponding organs, they indicate whenever an organ system is stressed or ill. (Additionally, it should be mentioned that we have similar systems of reflex zones in our hands, face, ears and eyes, as well as in our nose, on our head and in our back.) The reflex zone system of the feet, however, is not only the best known and most widely used area of its kind, but also one of the simplest and most clearly defined. Traditional therapy of the reflex zones of the feet consists of a special pressure point massage. A great many books with schematic diagrams of the reflex zones are available, so we will not pursue this aspect in any further depth.

It may be new to those interested in reflex zone massage that each of the seven chakras has its own individual "zone" in the feet and that the chakras can be influenced by massaging these points.

At first we were completely amazed by this easy yet highly effective method of harmonizing the chakras. With a few well-directed movements of our hands we were able to modify the chakra situation quite definitely. It is possible to massage one's own feet, but being massaged by somebody else is not only more effective, it is also more pleasant. Two people alternating in their treatment of each other is the ideal method. When we started massaging the chakra zones, we didn't know which technique to use, so we had to test various methods on different groups of people in order to determine their effectiveness. Here Bodo's ten years of experience with reflex zones and his practical knowledge of nearly all massage techniques proved to be very valuable.

As a result of our findings, we have found that a light and gentle form of massage using circular movements is best. In contrast to the well-known reflex zone massage, a lubricant, perhaps a mild cream, is also recommended.

We begin by massaging the reflex zone of the first chakra for about 2 or 3 minutes, which is quite sufficient. It should be remembered that chakra therapy does not function primarily on the physical plane, but on the energetic level. Therefore we do not require the force usually associated with reflex zone therapy. All we need to do is maintain a continuous and light physical contact while making circular movements with gentle pressure. The best way to do this massage is for the person receiving the massage to extend his feet toward the "masseur". While being massaged you should sit as comfortably as possible, or better still, lie on your back. The masseur should sit in such a way that he can easily reach the feet without straining. We found it most effective to simultaneously massage a chakra area on the sole of the right foot and the same area on the instep of the left, using a hand per foot. The procedure is then repeated the other way round, i.e. the respective chakra area is massaged on the instep of the right foot and on the sole of the left. We always make gentle, circular motions with one, two or three fingers, depending on the size of the area to be massaged.

However, we do not wish to limit you to a rigid massage procedure. What is really important is for the masseur to gently treat the areas of the individual chakras on the sole and the instep simultaneously for two to three minutes, reversing the procedure afterwards
In this manner we treat all of the seven chakra reflex zones in sequence. The masseur should concentrate on the chakra being treated, and the

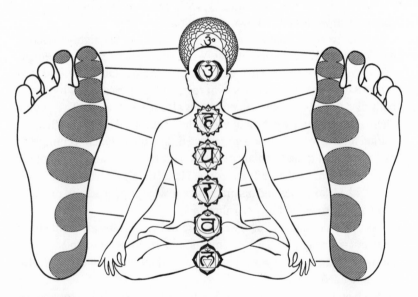

Right foot   Left foot

160

pressure of his fingers should be pleasant and appropriate. The person being treated should either relax completely or concentrate his attention on the chakra in question.

In our test groups we consistently found that the effectiveness of this therapy is intensified when we massage the individual chakra reflex zones in the same direction that they rotate. In other words, when we treat a man, we massage the first chakra in a clockwise direction, the second counterclockwise and the third clockwise, etc., while the opposite applies in a woman. (The rotational direction of the chakras is described in the chapter titled "The Purpose and Functions of the Chakras"). This procedure seems to result in optimal stimulation and harmonization of the energy flow. In some cases we have found that during the massage or afterwards, certain healing reactions known from other forms of therapy, such as slight detoxification, set in. Such reactions should not be mistaken for new symptoms of ill-health. Occasionally we also experience emotional release in the form of laughter or weeping. Reactions such as these should in no way be suppressed because they represent a physical self-regulating process and as such are important.

After a chakra massage has taken place, the "patient" should rest for a while. It can be extremely interesting to listen into our body during this quiet period. Has anything changed? How do I feel now? Am I balanced?

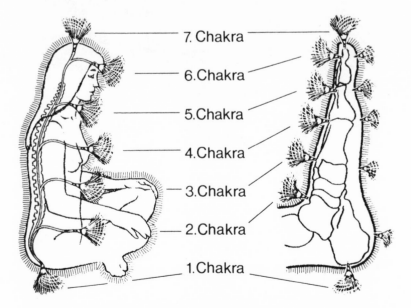

7. Chakra
6. Chakra
5. Chakra
4. Chakra
3. Chakra
2. Chakra
1. Chakra

The locations of the chakra reflex zones on the feet in relation to the body.
"As above, so below".

We have found that this therapy is most effective when repeated every second day in a series of seven treatments altogether. Naturally you can combine chakra reflex zone massage with any other method described in this book, whereby gemstone, color, aroma and sound treatment have proved most appropriate. Chakra reflex zone massage is also good and effective for infants and children. Many of the participants in our test groups have found it fun to do, and everyone was surprised by its far-reaching effects. A colleague of ours, Marianne Uhl, has published a book on this subject, titled *Chakra Energy Massage**. We would like to recommend this book to our readers, even though we do not agree with everything in it. This is because we never adopt a method for ourselves without having tried it out beforehand.

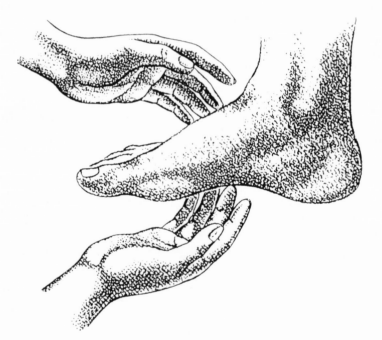

*) *Chakra Energy Massage*, by Marianne Uhl, Lotus Light Publications, Wilmot, Wisconsin, USA

Physical Exercises
for Releasing Blocked Energies

Keith Sherwood taught us the following exercises for loosening and releasing blocked chakra energies, and we would like to take this opportunity to thank him. He conducts excellent seminars on human advancement, harmonization and healing, and based these exercises on ancient knowledge of the Indian Yoga tradition.

These exercises immediately bring about noticeable beneficial and balancing effects to the entire organism. It is best to either lie down, sit with a straight back in the lotos position or sit on your heels. Now close your eyes and slowly drift into calmness. Your breathing should be relaxed and regular. Some practitioners like to slowly count backwards from 10 to 0 and sink into deeper states of relaxation with each digit.

Exercise One: Contraction of the Root Center
Exhale calmly and contract the pelvic area as strongly as possible by drawing the sphincter muscle inwards and upwards, as if trying to suppress a bowel movement. Now contract the genitals as far as possible, and draw in the lower abdomen in the area of the navel. This last step of the exercise supports the preceding contractions by pulling the rectum and genitals up and back.

When you have reached the greatest possible abdominal contraction, try to hold this position for a number of seconds before loosening and returning to the starting position. After resting for several seconds, repeat the three steps and the final state of contraction twice. Grant yourself several minutes of rest while retaining your consciousness in the area just contracted. This exercise will release blockages in the first and second chakras and stimulate the *kundalini* power. A feeling of rising energy and warmth usually follows the exercise and is perfectly normal.

Exercise Two: Contraction of the Diaphragm
(The diaphragm is a more or less horizontal sheet of muscle and sinews which separates the chest from the upper abdomen.) Continue to remain in a state of inner calm and relaxation, with your breathing as relaxed and as regular as before. Now exhale, and make an effort to raise your diaphragm up towards the chest. In doing so, try to press the organs of the upper abdomen towards the spine. Try and hold the contraction for several seconds and then loosen it. After resting, repeat the procedure.

While you rest, your attention should remain fixed on the part of the body you have just worked with. Generally, a vibrating feeling will set in, and some people may experience warmth or even heat. This reaction occurs when the solar plexus chakra is charged with energy.

Part of the energy released by this exercise rises up to the heart chakra, thus activating it. If you remain completely relaxed and concentrate on what is going on inside you, a feeling of deep inner peace will spread through you.

After several minutes of deep relaxation, move on to the next exercise.

Exercise three: Contraction of the Neck
Breathing through the nose, try to draw in and press down your neck by raising your shoulders and making your neck shorter. Remain in this position for several seconds and concentrate on the area of your neck. Relax and loosen it. Repeat the complete cycle three times and then relax for a while.

This exercise loosens blocked energies in the throat chakra and purifies this important channel between the head and heart. When the energy is able to flow freely again, an intense "glowing" feeling will be experienced in the area of the neck and shoulders, accompanied by a consciousness of inner strength, sincerity and self-confidence. These exercises harmonize the energies of Yin and Yang.

If you do these three exercises one after the other, you will experience an immediate improvement in your entire state of being. You should, however, take care not to overdo it. Doing these exercises once in the morning and once in the evening will be quite sufficient for the start.

As you gain experience, you can do the exercises several times in a row, but always remain aware of how you feel. Never go beyond your natural, inner limits. They will always let you know when it is time to stop.

These exercise have become a permanent part of everyday life for many people, including ourselves, as they only require a few minutes' time and yet achieve so much. Remember, it is not your theoretical knowledge of these highly effective exercises that lets you advance, but rather the practise of them on a daily basis.

Transmission of Universal Life Energy

The space surrounding us is filled with *prana*, the universal energy of life. It is therefore only logical to want to utilize and apply this highly effective cosmic energy in a direct and specific manner. We have already described one way of doing this in the chapter on chakra breathing. However, there are some other interesting and extremely effective methods that utilize this energy to both loosen blockages and further holistic development. One of them is called "Reiki".

This natural and holistic method of therapy was (re-)discovered around the middle of the 19th century by the Japanese doctor Mikao Usui, who travelled many Eastern and Western countries as a Christian monk. "Reiki" means "universal life energy" and is a form of therapy which transmits this cosmic, all-pervading energy to human beings. The therapist or person passing on Reiki merely functions as a sort of catalyst or channel. Without doing anything on his part, the cosmic energy simply flows through his hands into the client. Today, Reiki is one of the most rapidly spreading methods of healing. A number of years ago, we wrote a book about it called *Reiki - Universal Life Energy - Heals Mind, Body and Spirit - A Holistic Method Suitable for Self-Treatment and the Home, for Professional Practice and Teleotherapeutics/Spiritual Healing* which has appeared in several languages and been reprinted a number of times. Reiki has become so popular because it is easy to practise and yet highly effective. You can learn it in the course of two weekend seminars. During these seminars the ability to transmit energy is passed on from the teacher to the student in an initiation procedure which opens up the healing channels that exist in all human beings.

Reiki can even be practised by children, as it requires little in the way of specialized knowledge. This energy is endowed with a kind of "intelligence" of its own, meaning that it automatically flows to the area where it is needed in the correct dosage.

Today Reiki is being practised by hundreds and thousands of people all over the world, by laymen as well as medical professionals and healers. Reiki energy can be used to harmonize your own chakras and those of others.

Since Reiki energy flows through channels of healing which are natural to all human beings, it can - to a certain limited degree - be passed on by anyone who has begun to open up to the higher energies within him and around him. Even if you have not been through a Reiki initiation, if you have the feeling that your hands are capable of evoking calmness and relaxation, feel free to apply the following.

The practical application of Reiki to the chakras is fairly simple. You simply lay your hands on each individual energy center and let the harmonizing Reiki energy flow as it will.

Each of the seven chakras stands in a relationship of close interchange with some other one. Since Reiki energy flows through both hands at the same time, you can provide the chakras with life energy, and simultaneously harmonize and balance them by placing your hands on the chakras that exhibit a relationship to each other.

The seven-armed candelabra, a ceremonial and deeply symbolical artifact of the Old Testament and the Jewish faith, is an ideal illustration of the relationship of the chakras. Here the flames represent the chakras.

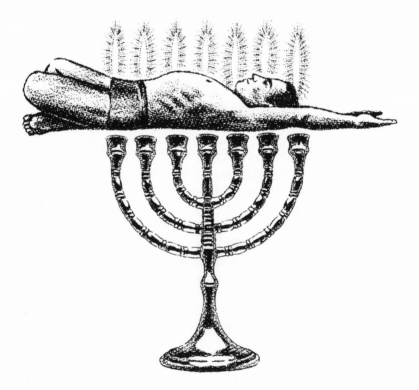

Seven-armed "chakra candelabra"

As can be seen, the central flame (the heart chakra, which has a central connecting function) maintains close contact with all of the other flames, or chakras. Many old traditions paid particular attention to the energy center of the heart, and if possible, we should always include it in all forms of treatment. We know from many people practising Reiki that they put both their hands on their heart chakra when they go to bed, often falling asleep in this position. If you wish to develop the qualities of the heart chakra, this is an ideal form of Reiki treatment.

In the illustration we can clearly see which chakras stand in relationship to each other, namely:

> the root chakra and the crown chakra;
> the sacral chakra and the inner eye chakra; and
> the solar plexus chakra and the throat chakra.

In order to bring the chakras into balance, simultaneously lay your hands on two related energy centers; for example, one on the root center and the other on the crown chakra; and so on. After having treated the six related chakras in pairs, use both hands to transmit Reiki energy to the heart chakra. In each case, keep your hands in place for three to five minutes. It is wonderful to silently observe the balancing of chakra energies.

In cases of problems or illness, it may also be useful to determine which chakras need charging with life energy. In the chapters on the individual chakras we have already described which chakras are related to the various parts of the body. Should we or a client of ours suffer from problems of the liver, a quick look at the list soon reveals that the liver stands in relation to the solar plexus chakra. We treat this chakra with the one hand and use the other to directly transmit Reiki energy to the liver. A further possibility is to treat the chakra related to the troubled one, thus letting Reiki balance out their energies. As we have seen, the heart chakra is the center of the entire system, therefore it is always advisable to balance out the heart chakra as well.

As this subject is only primarily of interest to Reiki practitioners, it shall not be discussed in any further depth here. We hope you have gained a little insight into the workings of Reiki, and recommend this form of therapy to everyone in search of a simple yet effective method of achieving all-round health and inner harmony.

Since many people in our culture tend to place more trust in technical devices than in nature's methods, some therapists employ a range of devices for treating patients with cosmic energy. In this respect, the use of model pyramids and orgone accumulators has proved to be of particular value.

The specific shape of a pyramid focuses cosmic energies and transmits them in a manner similar to Reiki, and so models are placed on the body to supply certain parts with energy. Today, a large variety of pyramids are available for this kind of treatment, all corresponding to the slope angle (51°) of the Cheops pyramid in Giza. For best results always make sure that one of the edges of the pyramid is aligned along a north-south axis. We have experimented with pyramids of various sizes made of wood, cast iron, marble, silver, copper, ceramic, aluminum, cardboard, synthetics and gemstones. We have always preferred working with pyramids made of rock crystal, rose quartz and amethyst, however, because we can incorporate them in gemstone therapy. As a rule, the pyramid is placed on the part of the body you wish to influence for five to ten minutes. The chakras react very positively to energy focussed in this manner. As in the other forms of therapy described here, it is recommended to direct your consciousness to the area being treated.

In his recently published book *"Die Glückspyramide"*, pyramid researcher Manfred Keppeler reports an interesting discovery. In the course of long investigations and calculations, he discovered that the angle of the Cheops pyramid is optimal for Egypt, but not for our part of the world, coming to the conclusion that the ideal angle for European countries should be 65° and not 51°. Pyramids constructed at this angle entail a considerable increase in energy potential (see Bibliography).

The orgone accumulator widely used in natural healing is another device we would like to mention without going into too great detail. It was designed by the scientist and psychoanalyst Wilhelm Reich (1897-1957), who in extensive research attempted to verify the "Odic Power" posited by Baron von Reichenbach (1788-1869) and find a practical use for it. Superficially, the orgone accumulator looks like a crate or cabinet. Its walls, however, consist of a number of layers of different materials assembled according to exacting specifications. The cabinet concentrates cosmic energies which are then put to therapeutic use. As a rule, the patient is seated inside the cabinet for a while to charge up with cosmic energy, a process which also energizes the chakras. Another method is to charge cotton balls in the orgone accumulator and then place them on the chakras or affix them with adhesive tape. As the kineological arm test described earlier has shown, this method proved to be surprisingly effective in several cases (see Bibliography).

If one (or more) of the methods described here appeals to you, try it out, and let yourself be surprised.

An Inner Journey
Through the Chakras

The journey we will now be describing is a form of guided meditation that will open the door to inner images and experiences. We not only quote the text here, but have also recorded it with suitable background music especially for this purpose (An English version is presently in preparation and will become available in the course of 1991. For details, please write to Windpferd Publications, 8955 Aitrang Germany). You can also record it yourself or have your partner or a friend read it to you. It should be read slowly, with short breaks between the sentences and longer pauses where indicated by a series of periods. Go on the journey with your friends. It will be wonderful to be able to share your experiences afterwards.

The journey is described in such a way that you can select individual passages if you only want to work on a specific chakra. Whatever the case, you should always observe your breathing at the beginning, and at the end allow yourself some time to reflect on what you have just experienced. The gentle fragrance of an aroma lamp or a joss stick, or the vibrations of gemstones can also accompany you on this journey. If you are not using our cassette, you might want to intensify the experience with soft background music.

Take care to ensure that you will not be disturbed during the entire course of the meditation. The room should be pleasantly warm and a handy blanket may also prove useful. Lie down comfortably and do not cross your legs, as this will impair the free flow of energy. (This does not apply to the lotus position, however.)

The following meditation will provide for a gentle opening and stimulation of the chakras. This will happen quite spontaneously, almost by itself. Since no effort on your part is needed, you don't have to do anything. Do not *try* to experience the images and sensations which will be suggested. Just relax and allow yourself to become sensitively aware of all ideas, thoughts and feelings that may come up while listening. Don't take an intellectual approach to the text either, since it will be acting on a completely different level of your being. Remind yourself of this inner attitude every time you are about to embark on this journey.

In the course of your inner journey you may experience previously restricted energies being released. Repressed emotions and feelings may arise to conscious awareness. Accept whatever happens. Do not reject anything. Surrender yourself to the natural healing power working within you.

Now lie down comfortably and close your eyes. With each outbreath you become more relaxed, sinking deeper and deeper into a state of calmness and inner peace ...

● Now allow your awareness to move to the first energy center located between the anus and sexual organs and opening downwards. Let your awareness linger there for a while without intent or purpose, without expectations. Your awareness gently stimulates your root chakra ot its own accord. You sense a slow and constant circulating motion, a warm flow of pulsating energy. From the center of this flow a clear, deep red light starts to emerge. In pulsating waves your first chakra emits its energy into your body, your blood carrying it into each and every cell, enriching them with peaceful warmth and vitality. Completely surrender to this pulsating stream of quiet power within yourself ...

Now you sense that your root chakra is opening up more and more, allowing the fresh and vital energy of the Earth to enter your body. Follow this energy to its source, deep down into the core of the earth, which is glowing in the same intense red light as your own root chakra. A continuous stream of energy rises from the innermost heart of Mother Earth, penetrating through the different layers. It flows into your body through your first chakra. You experience the hidden power dwelling within the Earth ...

Your own body was formed by this power and is constantly sustained and nourished by it. It is the very same energy that formed the contours of our planet, that gave birth to the countless plants, animals and human beings on Earth. You are intimately connected to the earth and her creatures. The same life force that permeates them is at this very moment pulsating through you. Sheltered within the cycles of the living Earth, you surrender to her protecting, nourishing and healing energies ...

Once this inner journey is over, you will remain in contact with this source of inexhaustible life energy incessantly streaming into your root chakra. Your stance in life is calm and composed, and you will be filled with gratitude and love for this wonderful planet, your home.

● While the pulsating power of the Earth continues to flow through you, let your awareness gradually drift to the sacral chakra. Located about a hand's breadth below your navel, it open forwards. Simply become aware of this area without expectations, without purpose. Your awareness stimulates your second chakra. You sense a subtle circulating motion, more vivid in its flow than the one in the root chakra. It feels like swirling warm water, a revolving and dancing motion of flowing energy. At its center a clear orange light starts to grow. It intensifies with every turn of the circulating flow. Its waves unfold, filling your body in ever-widening circles. They merge with the circulation of your blood and the purifying stream of your lymphatic system. Your body is now a single flow of living energy ...

And still the flowing energy expands, passing through the pores of your skin, surrounding and enfolding you, bathing you in its gentle strength. It sustains you playfully, caressing you, gently rocking you as if you were its child. You surrender into the caressing and rocking motion of this water of Life. Body and soul untie their knots, absorbing increasing amounts of purifying and enriching life force. Blocked channels open up, forgotten memories and feelings awake. From every direction new life flows towards you, filling you with its streaming energy ...

And still the vibrant flow of Life expands, growing into a boundless ocean of tender warm water, lovingly supporting and rocking you. Above you behold the dome of the sky. On the horizon rises a glorious morning sun, flooding sky and ocean alike with its golden-orange rays. You feel as if you have awoken to the very first morning of a new world. Waves of bliss arise within you, sweeping over the whole range of Life, touching everything and every being that has ever been created. In a deep and intimate way you know that the same engendering force of Life which is flowing through all of Creation is also flowing through you. The Life within you begins to merge with the Life of all. Full of confidence you surrender to its flow ...

Once this journey is over, you will remain in contact with this source of Life within you forever. You will be open to the generating and receptive powers of Creation, to the miracle of Life flowing within you and surrounding you.

● While the water of Life continues to flow through you, filling body and soul, you now let your awareness wander to your third energy center. Located a couple of inches above your navel, it opens forwards. Let your awareness linger there for a while without purpose or intent. Your awareness gently stimulates your solar plexus chakra, the source and base of your personal power. Whatever its present condition, you accept it as it is. Your acceptance allows your third chakra to relax more and more ... It starts to turn in a circulating flow of warm energy. Soon the circling motion allows a yellow golden light to emerge from its core. Like the light of the rising sun, its radiance increases, filling your body ever more with its soothing glow. Golden warmth touches you from within. Completely relaxed and at ease, you surrender to this golden radiance. Its light reaches down to the most unfathomable depths of your soul and fills them with brightness and clarity. Shadows and tensions dissolve. From the center of your body the illuminating light permeates the whole of your being until only peace, strength and abundance abide within you ...

The golden rays from within radiate out, enfold you in a ring of shimmering light and reach out into the world. Your third chakra has turned into a sun of utmost brilliance. It has come to be an inexhaustible source of Life-giving warmth, of power and light ...

When you return from this journey, you will organize your life from your inner center, from this center of light, peace and energy. The light within you will radiate out into the world, attracting abundance and light on all levels of being. You accept that you are a center of radiance for the plants, animals, human beings and everything else surrounding you.

● While the warm radiance of your inner sun still permeates you, let your awareness gradually wander to your fourth chakra. Level with your heart in the center of your chest, it opens forward. Simply notice this area, without expectations, without purpose or intent. Your awareness stimulates your heart chakra. You sense a most gentle, soft vibration which gradually manifests in a rose-colored sheen surrounded by an aura of radiating green. It feels like a tender blossom made of light, embedded in a ring of transparent leaves.

At the core of this blossom, the energy gently starts to circulate. While softly focussing your awareness on this motion, you sense how the blossom is opening up more and more, becoming a flower in full bloom. A loving vibration radiates from the open flower of your heart, delighting you all around with its touch of love and harmony. You feel as if you are carried by the hands of an angel, feeling completely understood in your deepest longing for love. You gladly surrender to this loving kindness and empathy ...

From the center of your heart you sense a deep joy welling up, a smile, an inner contentment. It feels like wonderful soothing music. Its waves spread throughout your body, awakening it to its own melody. They ring deeply into your soul, permeate it with love and harmony. They fill the space around you, reaching into the depths of Creation ...

And from all around, like an answer, music resounds, merging with the music of your heart into a perfect symphony. It opens the door to a new level of reality: you realize that a vibration of love and joy permeates each and every manifestation of Life. In accord with all of Creation, you vibrate in this music of all-pervading Divine Love ...

When you return from this journey, you will never be alone again. Through your heart chakra you will always be united with the innermost being of all things.

● While the music of your heart still resonates within you, let your awareness wander to your throat chakra, which has an opening towards the front and a smaller opening towards the back*. Just notice this area without expectations, without purpose or intent. Your awareness stimulates your throat chakra. The subtlety of its frequency gives rise to a translucent light-blue radiance. It is the vibration of the blue expanse of the sky. You now allow this radiant bright vibration to expand, filling the whole of your being ...

Life within you is expanding and brightening ever more until you become unlimited like the sky. You accommodate whatever exists in your inner and outer world, just like the infinite space allows for the life of all star, planets and suns to exist. Now you allow the dance of Life to unfold within the wondrous infinity of your own being ...

You accept everything as it is, you let everything come and go. In this infinite freedom of consciousness you are whole and complete. A bright wave of bliss vibrates through the unbounded space within you. There is stillness inside. You are completely quiet, listening to the infinity of space. You allow yourself to become a channel for all messages received by your innermost soul ...

When you return from this journey, you will continue to carry the bright expanse of the sky within you. The more you totally accept yourself, the more you will be able to let the energies stream out of you freely.

● While clear bright infinity continues to unfold within you, let your awareness wander towards the chakra of the third eye. Located slightly above and between your eyebrows, it opens forward. Just notice this area without purpose or intent. Your awareness stimulates your third eye chakra. You sense a silent circulating vibration. From within this silent motion a deep indigo-blue light starts to emerge, gradually becoming more intense. It is the light of a clear night with its secret life hidden in the infinity of space. Let your awareness enter this light, let your consciousness be ever more permeated by its silent luster ...

The vibration of the indigo-blue light makes you receptive and calm. Deeper and deeper you venture into this calm and quiet blueness. The silence within you grows. Thoughts are left behind. The whole of your consciousness is saturated by the peaceful rays of this silent light. On this

---

The opening towards the back belongs to a small subsidiary chakra which we have included here with the throat chakra.

deep level of being you are connected with the Universal Spirit, operating within you as within all Creation. You are opening yourself to boundless knowledge of cosmic intelligence, dwelling beyond all concepts and thoughts ...

When you return from this journey, you will go through life with increased awareness, silent openness and understanding of the truths hidden behind the external appearance of all the world's phenomena.

● While deep receptive silence continues to vibrate within you, let your conscious awareness now wander to your crown chakra. Located in the center of your cranium, it opens upward. Let your awareness linger there for a while without purpose or intent. Your attention ever so slowly and softly opens this gate, revealing a bright, clear, purple light. It is as if you enter a sacred realm, a temple of purple light open above. And through this opening a new, brilliant white light encompassing the whole range of colors floods down, filling the purple temple. Like a shower its blessings pour down on you. Every pore of your being opens itself to receive it, until every pore of your being opens up, absorbing the brilliant light until you are completely saturated. ...

This light knows no boundaries nor time. You realize that it has never ceased to glow within you as within the innermost heart of all Creation. In this perfect light you are one with the omnipresent Divine Being. While it vibrates in total silence, this light contains all music. Though quiet like the moment before sunrise, it contains the dance of Life in all its infinite steps and variations. Allow yourself to rest in this light, freed of all wishes and needs. This is your home. You have reached the goal of your journey ...

From now on part of this light will always shine within you. Accept that its glow radiates through your life and your world.

While the brilliant lustre of this clear white light still permeates you, let your awareness again turn to your crown chakra. You experience now how the colorless light transforms itself into the vibration of a bright clear purple. Let your awareness proceed to the chakra of the third eye. Here you experience how the colorless light transforms itself into the vibration of a deep indigo-blue.

Let your awareness continue to wander to your throat chakra. You now realize how the pure colorless light is turning into a light-blue vibration. Let your awareness drift further down to your heart chakra. Here you experience the colorless light transforming itself into a soft rose color and a clear, rich green.

Gently guide your awareness to your solar plexus chakra. Here you realize how the bright colorless light is turning into the vibration of a radiant gold.

Let your awareness wander towards the chakra of your sacrum. Here you experience the transformation of the colorless light into a vibration of bright orange.

Now move on to your root chakra. Here you experience the colorless light transforming itself into the vibration of a clear deep red.

Allow yourself to rest for a while in the wholeness of the colored vibrations of the colorless light, connecting you with the totality of Life. After returning from this journey the wholeness, the strength, the light and love which you have experienced will remain with you and continue to live within you, enriching you and your world. Allow it to happen of its own accord.

● Now direct your attention completely to your body. Take deep breaths and exhale deeply. Stretch your limbs and your torso a few times until you feel that you are back in the present moment. Give yourself some time before you slowly open your eyes.

Whenever you feel like it, you can take another journey, but give your soul time to digest and integrate these experiences. Each journey will be slightly different. If you practise regularly, your experiences will become deeper and clearer in the course of time and will become more and more part of your everyday life.

Appendix

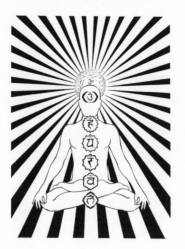

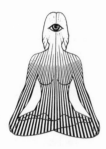

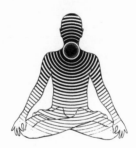

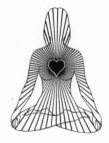

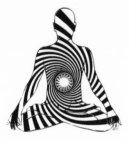

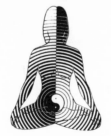

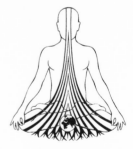

Chakras and Associated Factors

Chakra	Name	Symbol	Location
1st Chakra	Muladhara Chakra, Root Center, Base Chakra or Coccyx Center (root support)	4-petaled lotus	Between anus and genitals, connected to coccyx, opens downward
2nd Chakra	Savadhisthana Chakra, Sacral Chakra or Cross Center	6-petaled lotus	Upper part of sacrum, approximately at upper limit of pubic hair, opens forward
3rd Chakra	Manipura Chakra, Solar Plexus Chakra, or Navel Center, Spleen, Stomach, Liver Chakra	10-petaled lotus	Two fingers above the navel, opens forward
4th Chakra	Anahata Chakra, Heart Chakra or Heart Center	12-petaled lotus	Center of chest (breastbone), opens forward
5th Chakra	Vishuddha Chakra Neck or Throat Chakra or Communication Center	16-petaled lotus	Between inner collarbone and larynx, opens forward
6th Chakra	Ajna Chakra, Brow Chakra, Third Eye, Eye of Wisdom, Inner Eye Chakra or Command Chakra	96-petaled lotus (2 x 48 petales)	One finger above the nose center of forehead, approx. two fingers deep in head, opens forward
7th Chakra	Sahasrara Chakra, Crown Chakra, Vertex Center or 1000-petaled lotus	1000-petaled lotus	Center of top of head, opens upward

Chakras and Associated Factors

Chakra	Basic principle	Sensory function	Color
1st Chakra	Physical will to be	Smell	Fiery red
2nd Chakra	Creative reproduction of being	Taste	Orange
3rd Chakra	Shaping of being	Sight	Yellow - golden yellow
4th Chakra	Devotion, self-abandon	Feeling	Green, pink, gold
5th Chakra	Resonance of being	Hearing	Light blue
6th Chakra	Knowledge of being	All senses including extrasensory perception	Indigo, also yellow and violet
7th Chakra	Pure being		Violet, white, gold

Chakras and Associated Factors

Chakra	Astrological signs and planets	Associated gemstones	Element
1st Chakra	Aries / Mars, Taurus, Scorpio / Pluto, Capricorn / Saturn, (in Ayurvedic teachings: the Sun)	Agate, bloodstone, garnet, red coral, ruby	Earth
2nd Chakra	Cancer / Moon, Libra / Venus, Scorpio / Pluto	Carnelian, moonstone	Water
3rd Chakra	Leo / Sun, Sagittarius / Jupiter, Virgo / Mercury, Mars	Tiger´s eye, amber, yellow topaz, citrine	Fire
4th Chakra	Leo / Sun, Libra / Venus, Saturn	Kunzite, emerald, green jade, rose quartz, pink tourmaline	Air
5th Chakra	Gemini / Mercury, Mars, Taurus / Venus, Aquarius / Uranus	Aquamarine, turquoise, chalcedony	Ether (Akasha)
6th Chakra	Mercury, Sagittarius / Jupiter, Aquarius / Uranus, Pisces / Neptune	Lapis lazuli, indigo sapphire, sodalite	
7th Chakra	Capricorn / Saturn, Pisces / Neptune	Amethyst, rock crystal	

Chakras and Associated Factors

Chakra	Associated parts of the body	Associated glands	Associated hormones
1st Chakra	Everything solid, spine, bones, teeth, nails, legs, anus, intestines, prostate gland, blood, cell multiplication	Suprarenal glands	Adrenalin, noradrenalin
2d Chakra	Pelvic area, reproductive organs, kidneys, bladder, all liquids, such as blood, lymphatic fluid, digestive secretions, sperm	Reproductive glands, ovaries, prostate gland, testicles	Estrogens, testosterone
3d Chakra	Lower back, abdominal cavity, digestive tract, stomach, liver, spleen, gall bladder, autonomic nervous system	Pancreas (liver)	Insulin (gall bladder)
4th Chakra	Upper back, heart, rib cage and chest cavity, lower lungs, blood, circulatory system, skin, hands	Thymus gland	Thymus hormone (as yet scientifically unresolved)
5th Chakra	Lungs, bronchials, esophagus, vocal chords, throat, nape of neck, jaw, jowls	Thyroid gland, parathyroid gland	Thyroxine
6th Chakra	Cerebellum, ears, nose, sinuses, eyes, part of the nervous system, face	Pituitary gland (Hypophysis)	Vasopressin (antidiuretic hormone of the hypophysis
7th Chakra	Cerebrum, cranium	Pineal gland (epiphysis)	Serotonine (entaramine)

Chakras and Associated Factors

Chakra	Form of Music	Vowel	Tone
1st Chakra	Strongly rhythmic, (stomping beat)	"oh"	C
2nd Chakra	Flowing music, (folk dances, dance music)	short "o"	D
3rd Chakra	Fiery rhythms, orchestral compositions	long "o"	E
4th Chakra	Classical music, New Age music, sacral music	"ah"	F
5th Chakra	Overtone music and song, sacral and meditative dance, New Age music, reverberating sound	"eh"	G
6th Chakra	Eastern and western classical music, the sounds of cosmic spheres, New Age music	"ee"	A
7th Chakra	Silence	"m"	H

Chakras and Associated Factors

Chakra	Mantra	Nature experience	Associated aromas
1st Chakra	L A M	Dawn, sunset, fresh soil	Cedar, clove
2nd Chakra	V A M	Moonlight, clear water	Ylang-ylang oil, sandalwood
3rd Chakra	R A M	Sunlight, field of rape in bloom, ripe wheat field, sunflowers	Lavender, rose-mary, bergamot
4th Chakra	Y A M	Untouched nature, blossoms, pink sky	Rose oil
5th Chakra	H A M	Blue sky, reflections of the sky in water, gentle waves	Sage, eucalyptus
6th Chakra	K S H A M	Nightime sky	Mint, jasmine
7th Chakra	O M	Mountain tops	Olibanum, lotus

Chakras and Associated Factors

Chakra	Theme / Lesson	Female chakra spin direction	Male chakra spin direction
1st Chakra	Primal vital energy, primal trust, relating to Earth and the material world, stability, the power to succeed	left	right
2nd Chakra	Primal feelings, flowing with life, sensuality, eroticism, creativity, awe and enthusiasm	right	left
3rd Chakra	Unfolding of personality, working on feelings and experience, shaping one's being, influence and power, strength and plenty, wisdom, growing out of experience	left	right
4th Chakra	Unfolding of qualities of the heart, love, compassion, sharing, heartfelt empathy, selflessness, devotion, healing	right	left
5th Chakra	Communication, creative self-expression, openness, expansiveness, independence, inspiration, access to the subtle levels of being	left	right
6th Chakra	Functions of recognition, intuition, development of the inner senses, mental powers, projecting one's will, manifestation	right	left
7th Chakra	Perfection, highest recognition through inner contemplation, union with the Universal Being, universal consciousness	left	right

Chakras and Associated Factors

Chakra	Form of Yoga	Positive Power	Modes of Sleep
1st Chakra	Hatha Yoga, Kundalini Yoga	Stabilizing, grounding	On stomach, 10 - 12 hours
2nd Chakra	Bhakti Yoga	Purifying, starts things to flow	Prenatal position, 8 - 10 hours
3rd Chakra	Tantra Yoga	Transforming, shaping, purifying	On back, 7 - 8 hours
4th Chakra	Karma Yoga	Opening, connecting	On left side, 5 - 6 hours
5th Chakra	Mantra Yoga	Communicating, transmitting	Alternatingly on right and left side, 4 - 5 hours
6th Chakra	Jnana Yoga Yantra Yoga	Recognizing	Deep and half-awake sleep, about 4 hours
7th Chakra		Transcending	Half-awake sleep only

Epilog and Thanks

In the conclusion to this book, we would like to point out that we have only employed a bare minimum of the vast and often confusing array of Sanskrit terminology that exists on the subject of chakras. This is because we believe that many of the aspects described can just as well be depicted in words we are familiar with.

We would now like to thank Klaus-Peter Hüsch, a graphics artist, teacher of meditation and close friend, who rendered the illustrations. He did this with great patience, knowledge and creativity, and was more than once prepared to adapt his drawings to our wishes. At the same time, we also owe our gratitude to the publishers for the painstaking work they have put into publishing this book.

No one would be able to base a book about chakras on his knowledge alone, simply because most of what we know about this subject stems from ancient traditions. For this reason, and because we wanted to present knowledge of the chakras in as complete and yet as practical a way as possible, we have drawn on a great many different sources.

We would therefore like to thank all the people who, in the course of many years, have passed on to us their knowledge in both written and spoken form, as well as those who have provided us with instructions on various methods, thus helping turn theory into practice. At the same time, we also owe our thanks to the many people who helped us test some of the newer methods for inclusion in this book.

Last, but most certainly not least, we owe a debt of gratitude to the teachers and masters of old who gathered this knowledge of the chakras and preserved it for later generations. It is to these teachers and masters that we dedicate this book. May its contents provide a source of practical help to many people on their path through life.

Audiocassettes and CDs

Baginski, Bodo J./Sharamon, Shalila, Merlin´s Magic, *Chakra Meditation, a journey into the energy centers*. Audiotape approx. 50 min. guided meditation and 50 min. music. Lotus Light, Wilmot, 1991

Marianne Uhl, Achim and Bernd Bauer, *Music for the Heart Chakra*, CD 30 min. specially composed for the heart chakra.
Lotus Light, Wilmot 1991

Marianne Uhl, Achim and Bernd Bauer, *Music for the Root Chakra*, CD 30 min. specially composed for the root chakra.
Lotus Light, Wilmot 1991

Marianne Uhl, Achim and Bernd Bauer, *Music for the solar plexus Chakra*, CD 30 min. specially composed for the solar plexus chakra.
Lotus Light, Wilmot 1991

Bibliography

Baginski, Bodo J./Sharamon, Shalila, *Reiki - Universal Life Energy*, LifeRhythm, Mendocino, U.S.A., 1988.

Cousto, Hans, *The Cosmic Octave*, LifeRhythm, Mendocino, U.S.A., 1988.

Jünemann, Monika, *Enchanting Scents,* Lotus Light Publications, Wilmot, U.S.A., 1989.

Klinger-Raatz,Ursula, *The Secrects of Precious Stones*, Lotus Light Publications, Wilmot, U.S.A.

Mandel, Peter, *Energy Emission Analysis*, LifeRhythm, Mendocino, U.S.A.

Pierrakos, Dr. John, *Core Energetics*, LifeRhythm, Mendocino, U.S.A.

Uhl, Marianne, *Chakra Energy Massage*, Lotus Light Publications, Wilmot, U.S.A.

ADDRESSES and
SOURCES of SUPPLY
Fragrances, Gemstones, Herbs
Books and Cassettes

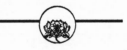

WHOLESALE
Contact with your business name,

resale number or practitioner license.

LOTUS LIGHT
Box 1008 CH
Silver Lake, WI 53170
Voice 414/889-8501 • Fax 414/889-8591

RETAIL
LOTUS FULFILLMENT SERVICE
33719 116th St, Box CH
Twin Lakes, WI 53181

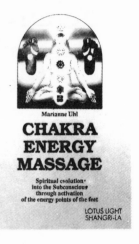
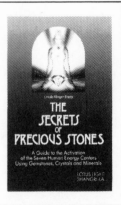